"If 'it takes a genius to make things simp[...]
its simple and easily accessible organi[...]
of complex patient presentations with clarity of principle and effective
methods. This book is destined to be a well-used reference in our
student clinic and classrooms as well as to promote 'genius' in treatments
professionally!"

—*Dr. Pamela Barrett, D.O.M.*—*Clinic Director of*
Southwest Acupuncture College in Santa Fe, New Mexico

"Skya Abbate's latest book belongs in the library of beginning
acupuncture students as well as seasoned practitioners. It begins with
the basics, but quickly dives deeply into more complex strategies to treat
common ailments that aren't always what they appear to be. Ms. Abbate
reminds us to always look below the surface and acknowledge the root."

—*Joanne Neville L.Ac.*

"Medicine is not magic nor miracle. It is a logical method of diagnosing
and implementing particular treatment strategies. As one of leading
educators in the field of Oriental medicine in America, Dr. Skya
Abbate accomplished another comprehensive guide full of important
information for those who learn and practice Oriental medicine. It
shines with her passion and wisdom."

—*Li Xu, D.O.M., Ph.D. (Acupuncture)*

"This book took me on an academic journey through the richness of
the foundations of TCM to the complexities of the patients with chronic
illness. Dr. Abbate eloquently reminds us of the necessary aspects of a
successful treatment from good rapport and atmosphere, to the deeper
levels of differentiating symptoms and treatment. Dr. Abbate writes with
humility and amazing systematic clarification. This is a wonderful book
for the budding acupuncturist! Simple, clear, concise, to the point!"

—*Corine Danchik B.S., M.S.T.C.M, L.Ac.,*
Academic Dean at Southwest Acupuncture College

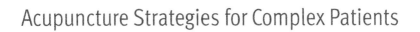

Acupuncture Strategies for Complex Patients

of related interest

The Living Needle
Modern Acupuncture Technique
Justin Phillips
ISBN 978 1 84819 381 9
eISBN 978 0 85701 339 2

The Fundamentals of Acupuncture
Nigel Ching
Foreword by Charles Buck
ISBN 978 1 84819 313 0
eISBN 978 0 85701 266 1

Intuitive Acupuncture
John Hamwee
ISBN 978 1 84819 273 7
eISBN 978 0 85701 220 3

Acupuncture and Chinese Medicine
Roots of Modern Practice
Charles Buck
ISBN 978 1 84819 159 4
eISBN 978 0 85701 133 6

Acupuncture for Body, Mind and Spirit
Peter Mole
ISBN 978 1 84819 203 4
eISBN 978 0 85701 155 8

ACUPUNCTURE
Strategies for Complex Patients

From Consultation to Treatment

Skya Abbate

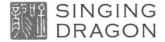
SINGING DRAGON

First published in 2019
by Singing Dragon
an imprint of Jessica Kingsley Publishers
73 Collier Street
London N1 9BE, UK
and
400 Market Street, Suite 400
Philadelphia, PA 19106, USA

www.singingdragon.com

Library of Congress Cataloging in Publication Data
A CIP catalog record for this book is available from the Library of Congress

British Library Cataloguing in Publication Data
A CIP catalogue record for this book is available from the British Library

ISBN 978 1 84819 380 2
eISBN 978 0 85701 336 1

Printed and bound in Great Britain

Dedication

To the graduates of the classes of 1988 through 2018 at Southwest Acupuncture College, Santa Fe, New Mexico for graciously giving me the privileged opportunity to teach these skills to you so that you may treat your patients in the authentic spirit of Chinese medicine.

Credits

Illustrations by Christine R. Oagley

Formatting of tables by Sandy Szabat

Other books by the author

Beijing: The New Forbidden City. Santa Fe, NM: Southwest Acupuncture College Press, 1991 and Summerville, SC: Holy Fire Publishing, 2009.

Holding the Tiger's Tail: An Acupuncture Techniques Manual in the Treatment of Disease. Santa Fe, NM: Southwest Acupuncture College Press, 1996.

The Art of Palpatory Diagnosis in Oriental Medicine. London, England: Harcourt Publishers, 2001.

Chinese Auricular Acupuncture. Boca Raton, FL: CRC Press, LLC, 2004.

Palpazione Diagnostica in Medicina Orientale. Turin, Italy: UTET Scienze Mediche, 2004. (In Italian)

Advanced Techniques in Oriental Medicine. Stuttgart, Germany: Thieme Publishing Group, 2006.

Bind Each Other's Wounds. Summerville, SC: Holy Fire Publishing, 2008.

The Catholic Imagination, Practical Theology for the Liturgical Year. Eugene, OR: Wipf and Stock, Resource Publications, 2012.

Communion, a desert story. Phoenix, AZ: Tau Publishing, 2013.

Creation, a fish story. Phoenix, AZ: Tau Publishing, 2013.

Incarnation, Daily Poems for Advent. Eugene, OR: Wipf and Stock, Resource Publications, 2013.

Visitation, a bird story. Phoenix, AZ: Tau Publishing, 2013.

Epiphany, an island story. Phoenix, AZ: Vesuvius Press, 2014.

Vesper, a horse story. Phoenix, AZ: Vesuvius Press, 2014.

Ascension, a swallow story. Phoenix, AZ: Vesuvius Press, 2015.

Chinese Auricular Acupuncture. Second Edition. Boca Raton, FL: CRC Press, LLC, 2015.

Wildflowers and the Call to the Altar. Eugene, OR: Wipf and Stock, Resource Publications, 2018.

Contents

Preface

Since 1988, I have taught this material along with diagnostic frameworks at Southwest Acupuncture College in Santa Fe and Albuquerque, New Mexico as one course out of four techniques courses offered at the college. In this new book, I have added more information about needling and its requisite diagnosis to make it stronger and more comprehensive thereby maximizing its use both as a college textbook and as a clinical manual for practitioners. A particular strength of this text is its user-friendly style, augmented with forms to assist the student/practitioner in organizing their diagnoses through treatment plans. I have noted these additions over the last thirty years and incorporated them into this book. Essentially, something seemed missing that students were not retaining, that is, the inextricable connection between diagnosis and needle technique and even more than that the importance of treating the fundamental essence of the patient over a symptomatic approach.

Through its clear and clinical pedagogy, in *Acupuncture Strategies for Complex Patients: From Consultation to Treatment*, I hope that the acupuncture practitioner recalls the richness and clinical applicability of the fundamental theories of Oriental medicine and how they can be applied to today's complex patients, many of whom suffer from chronic illness. Additionally, its allopathic treatment, in the case of pharmaceutical drugs, may consume the essential substances of the human body. Thus, this is a book for both the new or experienced clinician who is seeking effective, comprehensive treatment strategies to support the whole person in their foundational energies of *Qi, Blood, Jing, Jin-ye, Shen,* and *Marrow*. To these I add *Yin, Yang,* and *Zang-fu* energies.

The information presented herein is a synthesis of three experiences. Firstly, I undertook two China study tours specifically to accumulate knowledge about techniques that enhance therapeutic effectiveness. Secondly, I have used these techniques and adjunct therapies in private practice for over thirty years to personally assess their ability to treat the patient. Thirdly, I have taught these principles to over thirty classes of graduates in acupuncture college to ascertain without fail their continued success in treatment.

The first part of this book outlines what could be termed general treatment strategies that incorporate the infrastructure of Chinese medical treatment. These are thought processes and approaches to the practice of Chinese medicine for all conditions rather than for specific illnesses. I then take the reader from the philosophical underpinnings of Chinese medicine to the science and artistry of needle technique. Next, the book is devoted to various tonification techniques that strengthen the foundational energy of the patient. Finally, I cover techniques of dispersion sometimes needed for the treatment of secondary pathological products or cases of excess. In many chapters, actual case studies are included that illustrate the applications of the techniques presented. Clinical results are included for practitioners to assess their success in the treatment plans instructed in this work.

This book is by no means intended to be a needle technique nor a diagnostic compendium. Rather, it is a manual that can provide students and practitioners with useful treatment strategies. I have written this book to stimulate students, teachers, and clinicians to sharpen their diagnostic abilities and to coordinate their diagnoses with clinically effective techniques. Simultaneously, I hope to challenge the reader to go beyond the simple and sometimes automatic insertion of a needle, to consciously honing and bringing to full awareness the attention needed to skillfully and compassionately treat the complexity of the human condition through the foundational energies of the human person.

Skya Abbate, D.O.M. (Doctor of Oriental Medicine), Dipl Ac, Dipl C.H.,
M.A. Sociology, M.P.S. Pastoral Studies and M.A. Bioethics and Health Policy

Chapter 1

Building the Foundation, the Infrastructure of Treatment

Learning Objectives

The purpose of this chapter is to explore the nature of illness and the importance of diagnosis and prognosis in the treatment process. The clinical strategy is stressed on how treating the foundational energies of the human body is the root treatment to patient healing.

To practice medicine conscientiously demands a presence and integration of body, mind, and spirit on the part of the practitioner. Likewise, the practitioner needs to be healthy, physically strong, mentally astute, emotionally balanced, and spiritually oriented. Any practice, diet, lifestyle, meditation, exercise, or spiritual orientation the practitioner can adopt to cultivate a multidimensional approach to health is encouraged. As Abraham Herschel (Cohen 2010) reminded physicians in 1950 in his address to the American Medical Association, "To heal a person, you must first be a person."

Each type of healthcare has its own challenges. For instance, a Western physician needs to master appropriate diagnostic tests, drug interactions, and perhaps surgical skills. As a nurse, requisite knowledge encompasses proficiency with bedside manner and procedures. A massage therapist must cultivate skillful touch, anatomical discernment, and the real ability to feel a patient in their entirety. On the part of the Oriental medical practitioner, one's knowledge needs to extend beyond the familiarity of needle sizes and insertion depths, herbal properties, or prescription formulation. How to twirl a needle, assemble an herbal formula, or prescribe an antibiotic are skills in the arsenal of Oriental and Western medicine, and they must be taught and learned. While the ability to correctly diagnose and execute corresponding treatment plans with effective techniques is certainly integral to sound medical practice, the gift and necessity of connecting with patients completely, effectively, and genuinely is the benchmark of a true clinician in any tradition. So how can practitioners nurture this relationship with their patients?

In many books, generalized treatment strategies that address the whole person are absent as well as the logical thought processes that comprise the construction of treatment plans, order of needle insertion, and needling methods to name a few of the essential components that go into treatment strategies. These components are those that in essence support the foundational energy of the person, that is, their *Qi, Blood, Jing, Jin-ye, Shen, Marrow, Yin, Yang*, and *Zang-fu* energies.

The premise of my book, supported throughout and in its conclusion, is that the whole person must be treated in acupuncture medicine to maintain the integrity of Oriental medical philosophy, to preserve its lineage, but most of all to benefit the patient. This is a benchmark if not the cornerstone of Oriental medicine. Increasingly, as Chinese medicine adapts to Western culture, Chinese practitioners in China and acupuncturists in the West tend to treat from "a treatment of disease perspective," somewhat analogous to allopathic approaches, although broader than that lens. Much of what they do treatment wise is symptomatic for it is easy to get lost in the myriad symptoms of today's complex patients, especially those with chronic illness. While patients have diseases, their fundamental energetic substrates are what are disordered and require redressing. This is what I term their "foundational energies," that is, the basis of the human body viewed from an Oriental medical perspective. For students and practitioners who are developing their practices and are inundated with the avalanche of patient symptoms and complaints that are intrinsic to modern medical practice, the attention to a foundational style of treatment is not always given. Yet this approach is especially critical in order for the patient to heal and for the practitioner to establish sound habits in treatment.

The Chinese idea of treating the root, branch, and a combined root/branch are well-established Chinese approaches to treatment. The root is usually a deficiency and the cause of the symptoms that are called the branches. The patient generally presents at the level of the branches, that is, those acute symptoms that they are experiencing. It is easy to prefer to treat these multitudinous symptoms since they are the conscious level of patient complaint. Apart from recent trauma, or an acute attack of exogenous pathogens, or a flare up of root symptoms, the branches are usually linked to the root energies. Thus, a balanced treatment addresses both the root and the branch.

Pure branch treatments work best for recent or emergency type problems. Some claim root treatments take longer to treat and yield fewer results. Yet in my experience the skilled practitioner, who ascribes to a root approach as I do, has the expertise to see through the branches and to quickly get to the root. These ideas will become clearer as the strategies herein are explored. In essence, my idea of the foundational approach is a root treatment approach.

The comprehensive, foundational treatment of all life embedded in the essences of *Qi, Blood, Jing, Jin-ye, Shen, Marrow, Yin, Yang*, and *Zang-fu* energies leads to successful, meaningful, and long-lasting effective treatment for the patient. Treating the foundation does not mean that the patient will no longer be ill or injured, but it does mean that the patient is given the opportunity to recover through the restoration of right relationships between bodily energetics. But first we need to understand what is illness before we can intervene through treatment.

WHAT IS ILLNESS?

Human illness, with all its complex names and differentiations, ultimately wears the face of humanity. Illness is an integral part of life both personally and in the social setting of family, friends, and culture. It can manifest as a physical infirmity, a disability, psychological distress, an emotional difficulty, a spiritual affliction, financial stress, violence and abuse, social injustice, or a family problem. Illness is as fundamental to life as joy, sorrow, and all of the emotions and events that the human person can experience. The experience of illness can be shocking, surreal, and sorrowful. Hope and humor, compassion and communication, technology and tenderness, can help one cope with it. All are necessary tools in the treatment of disease. While illness is a natural part of life it is just as natural to want to help alleviate it. If people accept illness and its meaning, it has value, but admittedly one that is hard to appreciate in its throes.

WESTERN AND ORIENTAL VIEWS OF ILLNESS

A common Western definition of illness refers to a state of being sick or having an ailment and this is certainly an acceptable definition. But it is as equally certain to most people that there is a greater complexity to this state than is revealed through its definition for there may be multiple factors which cause and sustain an illness that manifest as the broken down aspects of the person.

Physiological theories about how the body works differ according to Western and Oriental viewpoints. Logically, treatment in any medical paradigm is intrinsically dependent upon the diagnosis or perspective from which it is perceived. For instance, there is a Triple Burner organ–meridian complex in Oriental medicine but there is no Triple Burner in Western medicine. Likewise, in Oriental medicine, the Spleen plays a major role in digestion, while it has no connection with digestion in Western science. So the philosophical paradigm is intrinsic to diagnosis and treatment.

Western doctors characterize illness according to two etiologies— as either organic or functional. An organic illness is one that is caused by an identifiable abnormality such as a knee disorder due to a torn ligament or a strep throat due to a bacterial infection. Organic illnesses have known etiologies and mechanisms called pathophysiology by which they normally progress if they are not treated. Western medicine is generally good in the treatment of those illnesses that have an organic etiology, for instance, in surgically repairing a torn knee ligament or prescribing an antibiotic for a sore throat due to a bacterial infection.

In contrast to an organic illness, a functional illness is one in which there is no objectively identifiable basis for the disorder, as in some varieties of insomnia or anxiety. Many times these illnesses are referred to as psychosomatic disorders, and the person is even labeled a hypochondriac if no cause can be identified for the complaint. Yet these patients' symptoms are no less real than those of the torn knee ligament or the sore throat; sometimes they are even worse. The person is frequently made to feel that they are exaggerating their complaint or that it is not real, thus leading to lack of treatment, palliative treatment, mistreatment, or an exacerbation of symptoms.

Oriental medicine as an energetic medicine does not make the distinction between an organic and a functional illness. The Oriental theory of the *Zang-fu* organs accounts both for the literal, discrete, physical problems of the body, that is its organic etiology, as well as its energetic or functional disturbances. Oriental medicine does not dichotomize a separation of the body/mind as does Western medicine, thus Oriental medicine assists in the complete, integrated care of the person. In this sense, Oriental medicine has an edge over most healthcare systems because it recognizes patterns of energy disturbance versus the symptoms. The body/mind/spirit are interdependent and treated as such.

Culturally, an organic dysfunction or a functional disease may be viewed by some as an event totally isolated from their lives. It is something that has "happened to them," or "gets them." It may even be an "act of God," as opposed to something that they may have had a direct, indirect, or even no role in creating. Patients may dismiss a whole range of ailments as being totally disconnected with their lives and consequent health. The illness may be viewed as something they cannot control, or it is due to contagion or genetics, or it is a problem that does not yet have a pill to cure it. The illness is rarely seen as other than physical even when it is intimately connected with the spiritual, mental, emotional, psychosocial self. The very fact that much illness is socially acceptable, for instance considered a legitimate reason for various behaviors such as absence from work or a social event, is further proof that illness is not perceived as related to the self, the mind, or the culture. We are inflicted with it. It is out of our control. For some patients, the illness defines their life's meaning and it is something they may actually cling to for a definition of themselves or their circumstances. They may not want to really get better as this will entail redefining themselves through new behavior.

The other side of the coin is that some patients feel that whatever illness they experience is one that they have directly created and so they are always looking for a causative factor to correct it. But much illness in today's complex, stressful, globalized, interconnected world is not understood or its causes identifiable, preventable, or controllable as they intersect or cannot be identified. Certainly if there are things patients can do to correct health disorders this is highly encouraged through self and patient education for life should be safeguarded whenever possible and patient education by the practitioner is critical in this regard. This is the highest calling of physicians—to teach patients and to promote life in all its forms.

Michael Greenwood, M.D. (1999, pp.51–52) writes in commenting on beliefs of the allopathic medical establishment, that the average patient desires to be fixed and the doctor thinks that only he can do it. He says,

> It is my view that when we are ill we are not helpless at all but rather deny our own power, willfully blinding ourselves to our own strength; and, further, that it is this blindness to our true nature that is ultimately what illness is. What our society as a whole cannot face—personal integrity and responsibility—individuals are compelled to grapple with when ill.

He continues,

> The power of the medical establishment is based on our collective insistence that the physician controls our sickness, as though it were a distinct and external phenomenon. Our fear of illness—our fear of loss of control—seems, paradoxically, to leave us craving a system that will corroborate our own denial of our power. But when we talk about our "power," we must be sure we know what we are talking about, for there is a very great difference between the *ability to control*, and the deep resources of *inner strength*—either of which can be termed "power." The abrogation of the ill individual's inner strength in the Western medical model of doctor-patient relationships seems clearly intended but it perhaps is not fully understood or acknowledged. Where has the power gone if we don't feel we have it? (p.52)

He offers us his insight into what he feels needs to be done on the individual's part to heal.

> Tackling such an apparently awesome power is central to healing. If the experience of illness makes us feel vulnerable and helpless—at the mercy of both the illness and the medical establishment—the healing

process must include a retrieval of power and a sense of being in control of our experience. While this idea may be attractive in theory, however, fear of "dis-ease" (pain or illness) is written into the very fabric of our psyches and of modern medicine. Our health care system seems to function on the implicit assumption that patients are helpless "victims" dependent upon the all knowing and all powerful doctor.

As a medical doctor he makes some good points about the cultural perception of illness, the power of the medical establishment, and the importance of the patient's inner strength in regaining power. This strength comes from the interpretation of the illness and how it is managed.

In the Orient, the Chinese, with over 5000 years of accumulated medical observations and treatment, perceived the body's processes and dysfunctions as being subject to certain natural phenomena. The basic definition of illness in Oriental medicine is that it is an imbalance between life energy that can be adjectively described as the *Yin* and *Yang*, or the Five Elements, the *Zang-fu* organs or other energetic interrelationships. In most cases illness is caused by the person not living in accordance and harmony with the natural law, for instance by not getting sufficient nutrition, sleep, and exercise, or by overworking. Holding on to emotions consumes, drains, weakens, or stagnates energy that then leads to imbalance or illness. Simply put, illness is life out of balance.

Oriental practitioners feel empowered by this definition of illness because imbalance implies that there is something positive and even measurable that can be aimed at, that is, balance. This is a different, positive view of health versus the Western definition of health as not being sick. However, experienced clinicians certainly know that just as imbalance can be redirected in many instances towards the positive image of ample *Qi* (energy) and *Blood* that creates health, so too they know that such balance can be precarious and not always possible to achieve. Additionally, that balance is relative to the person in regard to all their energetic components of *Qi*, *Blood*, *Yin*, *Yang*, and *Zang-fu* organs so one person's balance is different from another's. Yet there are common denominators as human foundational energies that are the same.

Because the Chinese see the human body as but *Yin* and *Yang*, with *Qi* and *Blood* being their material manifestations, when the *Qi* and *Blood* are ample and perform their associated physiological roles, the body is healthy, organ systems are harmonious, and the state of the organism is one of balance. If pathology exists in the *Qi* or the *Blood*, and ultimately their deepest basis, the *Yin* and the *Yang*, disharmony or imbalance results causing various signs and symptoms associated with the corresponding etiological factors. These patterns are consistent and identifiable for all humans.

Oriental medicine posits that two factors are always involved in disease—Evil *Qi* (*Xie Qi*) and the True *Qi* (Antipathogenic *Qi*). Evil *Qi* encompasses the concept of the causative factors of illness, that is, anything that causes illness is evil. There are four types of Evil *Qi*: the exogenous pathogens, the endogenous pathogens, the miscellaneous pathogens and the secondary pathological products.

The exogenous pathogens are the climates of wind, cold, damp, dryness, heat, and summer heat and the pathogens that mimic them such as viruses that produce common cold symptoms, or bacteria that produce heat symptoms like a bad sore throat. The endogenous pathogens are the emotions of anger, joy, fear, fright, grief, melancholy, and worry and all their numerous nuances. Both the climates and the emotions can cause *Zang-fu* organ disharmonies, as well as be a product of their dysfunction. For instance, weak Kidney energy can make one fearful or weak Lung function allows wind to enter the body and allergies to develop.

The miscellaneous pathogens are a type of Evil *Qi*. They include lifestyle variables including food consumption, exercise levels, drug use, trauma, sexual activity, and other factors connected with lifestyle. Finally, the secondary pathological factors of Damp, Phlegm, and Stagnant *Blood* are dually complicated causative factors of illness because they are physical pathological products that have developed as a product of *Zang-fu* organ dysfunction. In these cases there are two problems to treat—the organ dysfunction and the physical product of Damp related entities or Stagnant *Blood*. As such, these illnesses are more difficult to treat.

In contrast to Evil *Qi*, the True *Qi* pertains to the proper functioning of the body. True *Qi* is a product of the healthy interrelationship of all the organs and their physiological materials, what we might call in Western medicine our immunity. When the True Qi of the body is intact, then evil winds and spirits will not be able to penetrate, so say the Chinese classics, meaning immunity is in place and illness does not develop. The strength of the True Qi, a foundational energy, is always regarded as the most important variable affecting one's health. Its paucity is generally considered the leading cause of illness.

Ultimately then in Oriental medicine, much treatment can be directed around strengthening the True Qi or what I term the foundational energies of the body. However, there are times when the strength of the evil pathogen may be of such virulence that it overcomes the ability of the person to resist it and then disease results such as in the case of the flu, viruses, or the plague.

Oriental physicians Beinfield and Korngold (1998, p.80) beautifully express the notion of how illness arises. They say,

> Health and illness coexist and arise out of the same conditions. Disease doesn't come from nowhere—it emerges from a lived life. Simply put: Chinese medicine not only focuses on the content (the disease), but also on the context (the person who has it). Everyone exists within a matrix that includes a family, job, home, neighborhood, geographic area, and psychological and cultural milieus. Chinese medicine considers the impact of all these influences.

The task of the physician is to dissect the multifaceted diagnostic data revealed by the patient, and to arrive at an understanding of the causative factors of the person's illness or their patterns of interaction.

The condition of the world influences the person and many factors are to a large degree out of the immediate range of our individual control but have been caused by the species such as its contribution to global warming. The very fact that humans live in a physical and social world means that there will be a biological/environmental/social component to illness, and those elements cannot be ignored. They need to be acknowledged so that they can be addressed. This necessitates that physicians, by philosophical orientation, need to treat the whole person and to be willing to look at the wholeness of the person's life and to courageously inquire about it. While this is not an easy task, it is the physician's mandate to glean the proper conclusion about the person's life that enters into the etiology, diagnosis, pathophysiology, and treatment of disease. Without it, neither an appropriate treatment plan and useful patient education can be constructed, nor true lasting healing achieved.

On an even deeper level, acupuncturist and writer Lonny Jarrett (1998, p.315) knowingly acknowledges,

> If we accept the premise that attitudes, thoughts, and interpretations play a significant role in influencing health, then it becomes of primary importance to intervene therapeutically at the level of the patient's belief system.

He underscores my contention that the meaning of the illness needs to be interpreted and conveyed to the patient if the patient cannot decipher it. True healing begins at that point.

THE NATURAL CARE OF LIFE

Medicine is not magic nor miracle. It is a logical method of diagnosing the body based upon a particular theoretical framework and as a result implies particular treatment strategies. Many natural medicines, such as naturopathic and Oriental medicine, believe that examining the wholeness of life is necessary in order to comprehend the condition of the person. Those who maintain that "when you're sick, you're sick throughout" aptly understand this. Physical treatment and recovery may be less important than the social/spiritual meaning or experience of the illness.

Modern research is confirming what Oriental physicians have assumed for at least three thousand years: emotions, attitudes, thoughts, the "inner" life, all come together to create health or illness. Goleman (1991, p.13) claims,

> The belief that the human body is a little more than an extremely sophisticated machine has led, in the West, to many extraordinary advances; for example, the remarkable developments in surgery and drug therapy. Yet despite these spectacular successes, modern medicine generally fails to recognize that the mind and the spirit have an extremely powerful effect upon the body, and that the human body is more than the sum of its chemistry and mechanics.

Particularly if confronted with a disease that is difficult to cure, it is important to treat the mind rather than the body because changing the person's way of thinking about and managing the illness may be more effective than treating the disease directly.

Life is impermanent. But if a modus operandi or a mission statement acknowledges that human life extends beyond the material sphere, and practitioners treat what they see, do no harm, and do the best they can, it is hard to go wrong, especially if the patient's emotional cues as well as the bodily cries for help are heard. The spirit, the *Shen*, is amenable to intervention.

Spiritual factors include the sense of meaning, purpose, and values that are at the core of existence. It is easy to neglect the patient's *Shen* because its manifestation is somewhat less tangible than the realm of physical complaints. Yet in the clinical theater, to practice medicine fully, beyond textbooks and theory, demands this foundational perspective that the material and the immaterial have no borders.

Goleman (1991, p.11) agrees by citing that,

> This is not to imply that emotional distress outweighs biological factors in disease, or that psychological help can replace medical care. But the bottom line from these and other new studies seems to be that attending to patients' emotional distress along with ordinary medical care can add an extra margin of healing in many cases.

Medical doctor Larry Dossey (2002, p.12), in like manner, summarizes that, "To omit the spiritual element from our medical world view is not only narrow and arbitrary, it appears increasingly to be bad science as well." Further, in commenting on medical education in the United States, Thomas Kelting (1995) points out that the Western medical paradigm is not whole or balanced because it ignores spirituality and offers a mechanistic view of health and disease.

I ask: are we doing the same thing in holistic healthcare schools? What beliefs are we conferring to our students about the nature of health, healing, the recognition of the spirit, and the role of the doctor in the healing process? Are we teaching that herbs and the needle can treat everything? While the Oriental physician is more likely to address lifestyle factors and make dietary and exercise recommendations, how far are we willing to go to help our patient discover the beliefs, values, and emotions that may be linked to their illness? How can we best diagnose and treat our patients?

THE DIAGNOSIS

The purpose of the interview is to gather the most complete and accurate information about the person so that practitioners know how to diagnose and then treat the patient. All practitioners must acknowledge the patient's chief complaint; yet at the same time see the major complaint within the broadest context of the patient's life and medical history. Oriental medical practitioners, or those with a naturalistic bent, are at an advantage to discern the patterns of disharmony since they think holistically. In this way they gain the perspective on how the major complaint arose, what it is related to, and how it is progressing. Ideally they are not diagnosing symptomatic complaints but the entire person.

An accurate diagnosis is essential before treatment can proceed. A diagnosis, like a hypothesis, is an educated assumption about what is going on with the person. It is not a concrete label that circumscribes the life of the person. For instance, if from a Western point of view a person has allergies, in Oriental medicine that person is not just some-one who has allergies and as such should not be treated as a "disease " or an "allergy person." This is a pitfall that the allopathic world tends to accept. It sees the person within the very narrow perspective of a diagnostic label and treats the symptoms in a limited fashion with some consideration to other healthcare problems that they may have. Although there are some common denominators of symptoms that characterize allergies such as red eyes, sneezing, or stuffy nose, to lump all allergy sufferers together ignores the individuating aspects of the disharmony of each person.

Some students and even practitioners balk at this notion that the diagnosis is as fluid as a hypothesis and prefer that it is written in stone, but clinical experience bears out the educated guess nature of the diagnosis. Correctly, some doctors and healthcare providers are frequently at a loss to provide a definitive diagnosis. They change it based upon intervening time, in relation to diet, medications, and herbal formulas and therapies be it massage, physical therapy, acupuncture, laboratory tests, and a host of other reasons. This is the correct methodology—fluidity—for fluidity is the nature of energy.

In Oriental medicine, disease is differentiated, meaning it is individualized, based upon the person's complete symptom pattern. The language of the diagnosis is by nature succinct and precise, and should capture the essence of the person. For instance, a diagnosis might be Liver *Qi* stagnation due to Lung and Kidney *Qi* deficiency. Even though diagnostic terms are necessarily used, Oriental medical practitioners must not label patients in comparable Oriental medical language such as the Kidney *Yin* deficient person or with patient with stagnant Liver *Qi*. To do so is simply the same thing as a Western counterpart but with different terminology. The challenge of diagnosis is to be present in the moment to each patient and to treat the pattern of disharmony for that person, that is, what is the root and connections of the patient's Kidney *Yin* deficiency or stagnant Liver *Qi*.

Chinese scholars Claude Larre and Elizabeth Rochat de la Valle (1995) describe in their book, *Rooted in Spirit*, that the good practitioner's diagnosis is a connection from deep within himself to the spirits of the patient, which are showing signs recognizable to the practitioner. Thus he goes at once to the seat of the malady, which will be the place where he intervenes. The implication here is that the best diagnosis is not necessarily framed in the language of any diagnostic paradigm as described above, but gets to the primary, elemental, energetic or organ pathology with a swiftness derived from experience, observation, insight, and diagnostic acumen from even the slightest of microcosmic clues, what I call their foundational energy.

For instance, I remember when going to school of being told of a famous practitioner who stood at his corner office window and watched patients approach his office from the parking lot. The practitioner usually had the patient diagnosed before they entered the office! But, if not, he did so by the time the patient knocked on the door and he heard the way in which the patient knocked. This level of diagnosis is what Larre and Rochat de la Valle are referring to—that ability to get to the diagnosis with a swiftness derived from experience. Clinical experience and the ability to bring one's entire presence to diagnosis and treatment can make it as simple as that.

The concept of the diagnosis as capturing the essence of the person is very empowering by virtue of its fluidity. This does not mean that a diagnosis should be general, casual, haphazard, or incorrect.

The practitioner should always do their best to ensure the most accurate perception at the time. Reevaluating the diagnosis every time the patient is seen allows for that fluidity in diagnosis and treatment. The diagnosis is a springboard to the treatment plan that directs the point selection, needle technique, patient education, herbal remedies, Western medications, laboratory tests, or other aspects of patient care.

THE PROGNOSIS

After the diagnosis has been formulated, the patient must be informed of the prognosis, or the expected therapeutic outcome. Whether a diagnosis is framed in Oriental medical terms, or complex Western language, it is the job of the physician, nurse, physician's assistant, or other healthcare provider to make sure that the diagnosis is clear and understandable in ordinary language. For instance, do not tell the patient that they have Liver *Qi* stagnation or benign prostatic hypertrophy without explaining to the patient what that means. If constraint is felt in the pulse or a purple hue seen on the tongue, that means that the *Blood* and *Qi* are not flowing smoothly and are stagnating, thus giving rise to tension expressed in the wiry pulse, or the vascular impediment causing the purple tongue. That is also why they are feeling irritable or have a headache. As a healthcare provider you have spent years learning to understand these concepts and so you are able to convey the richness of your experience in simple language to the patient. Patients can understand and verify your explanations when you are present for them and you take the time to explain things to them, with patience, simplicity, and clarity.

It is critical to give the patient a sense of the likely therapeutic outcome, which is the prognosis. Sometimes the prognosis is serious or poor and it needs to be delivered sensitively. Other times it is just an energy disturbance like Spleen *Qi* deficiency, or a skin rash due to an irritant, a miscellaneous pathogen. However, as medical experts, it is one's ethical obligation to be honest with patients about their condition for this is why they have come for treatment. They need to receive an honest and accurate assessment of their health or life force. This is not to say that a healthcare provider cannot make mistakes, hence additional professional opinions are always an option and should be suggested if warranted. Because healing happens on many levels, there may be other treatment avenues that the patient may choose to pursue.

The way in which the diagnosis or prognosis is conveyed is critically important. A transfer of the simplest information can have healing or devastating powers. The healthcare provider is part of how a patient experiences their illness. As Konner (1987, pp.330–331) found in his medical education in observing his mentors in the treatment of terminal illness, "There was much to be learned from a healing voice and touch—laughter, gentleness and dignity, these gestures can be healing in almost every case. That is, they made a difference in the choices the patients made, in the way that they conceived of their futures, in the way they felt about themselves."

Keep in mind that healing is a process, not an isolated event in linear time and space. Healing is connected with its interpretation, its expectations, and the course of treatment. How the diagnosis and the prognosis are relayed is part of this healing process. Regardless of the prognosis or the personality of the patient, Lonnie Jarrett (1998, p.331) expresses this perfectly when he says, "It is imperative that with every communication with our patients that the practitioner reinforces the patient to create meaning in life that adds to rather than detracts from vitality." This may be difficult to do, but it should be a guiding principle when practitioners encounter their patients. As long as there is life, it must be nourished and cherished. It is not practitioners who heal or who can predict with certainty any therapeutic outcome. Healing moreover can come even in the midst of death, for it is the whole person who is healed, not just the physical body but also the integration of body, mind, and spirit. Illness and death are part of the natural law and acknowledging that gives purpose and direction to treatments, the physician's practice, and their patient's illness.

Summary

This paradigmatic perspective of diagnosing the foundational energies sets the stage for the actual clinical encounter and the infrastructure of eventual treatment. Its philosophy is encapsulated in the adage "To go against the roots is to attack the trunk and destroy authenticity itself" (Larre and Rochat de Vallee 1995, p.135).

Chapter 2

The Interview, the Heart of the Clinical Encounter

Learning Objectives

In this chapter, the fundamental importance of the interview as a leading method of diagnosis is explored as a veritable window to the soul of the patient, so that treatment may be planned.

In any medical tradition, the interview is the heart of the therapeutic clinical encounter. In Oriental medicine and most healthcare systems, it is standard in varying degrees to ask the preliminary questions about the major complaint, accompanying symptoms, onset and duration, and family and personal medical history. Additionally, as students and practitioners of Oriental medicine know, asking the many detailed physiological questions known as "the Ten Questions" has become the foundation of the Oriental medical intake. Through these voluminous questions we can gain a view into the fullest context of the patient's life and health. For the most part, as Oriental medical practitioners, we do not do diagnostic tests ourselves such as lab work or x-rays although we may rely upon them for information, hence the importance of the interview is further emphasized.

A more holistically oriented healthcare paradigm incorporates questions that extend beyond the basics asked by allopathic physicians because they measure energy patterns in all the physiological systems. The person as a whole is interviewed instead of their medical complaints such as allergies or headaches.

In commenting on allopathic medicine, medical doctor Konner (1987, p.130) claims,

> It is often said that 85% of the information needed to make a diagnosis is in the history, with most of the rest coming from tests. This dictum has always made me wonder why so little emphasis in my medical training was placed on how to talk to patients, and I suspected that this was because so few doctors knew.

More than medical information is offered in the interview. As a narrative, information that is rich in etiological factors emerges. Respected nurse Mary Nagai-Jacobson (Nagai-Jacobson and Burkhardt 2002, p.19) states,

> Healthcare professionals who listen to your stories—those personal accounts of the events in our life—may learn much more than your medical history. Life stories provide the framework for relating complex thoughts and feelings that cannot be catalogued in a list of illnesses and treatments. What you choose to tell and how you choose to tell it convey your attitudes towards health and illness and may help your doctor help you. Stories are places to put facts so we can understand them better. They include interpretations that add meaning to the events of our lives. Telling and hearing stories enhance our understanding of others and ourselves. Stories told about illness and injury help us review these processes, insights and activities of our lives. By hearing about the events associated with our ailments, healthcare practitioners can facilitate our healing process. We release energy when telling a story, get things "off our chests", so we can get on with the business of healing.

If you listen to the patient's story, in addition to their major complaint, they will tell you what the problem is and what help they want. It may not be a prescription they want for their palpitations or any medical complaint but acknowledgment that they have been under extreme stress and now need to find a way to manage it, for instance, by thinking about how they can view things and changing that over taking a pill.

INITIAL AND FOLLOW-UP INTERVIEWS

The interview consists of two vital dimensions: the content and the spirit. Analysis of both is needed to gain information about the patient.

Unless one is conducting an emergency interview, which is more succinct, and indeed there are times to so do in any paradigm, there are basically two styles of interviews, the initial and the follow-up interviews. The initial interview is a long, detailed procedure that sums up the life experience of the patient at that point. It encapsulates the life span of the person. In Oriental medicine, it consists of the "Five Preliminaries" and the "Ten Questions." The Five Preliminaries concentrate on the major complaint and its onset, duration, differentiating characteristics, and family and personal medical history. The Ten Questions are made up of the numerous physiological questions that review the body systems such as body temperature, perspiration, energy level, digestion, absorption and elimination, reproduction, sleep patterns, pain, and emotions.

The follow-up interview is conducted on subsequent visits. It is relatively short and pertains to the major complaint, other active problems that were identified at the initial visit, and patterns of disharmony that are part of the patient's history, and any new developments. Both the initial and follow-up interviews have the same goal, that is, to learn as much as possible about the person's energetic state.

INTERVIEW SKILLS

The interview process discloses the state of the human spirit when it is conducted with an openness and rapport that allows the richness as well as the sickness of the person to emerge. "Chinese medicine trains you to develop yourself as an instrument. You don't keep your subjectivity outside the door. Use your senses and emotional responses to read the patient" (*Choices* 2002, p.19).

Although people like to talk about themselves, in most instances this does not automatically happen in the treatment room. Patients typically defer to the person they feel is in charge and that is you, the practitioner. Listening to the patient helps to diffuse that power differential. To obtain quality information, you and the patient must establish mutual rapport, a trust that leads to openness in communication. As the facilitator of the healing process, you need to work the hardest to make this happen. Rapport is almost sure to transpire if you are genuine in your dealings with the patient. Such authenticity on your part will open the door of trust.

Caring and trust come across in the warmth and clarity of your voice, and the intelligence and coherence of the interview during which time the patient assesses your dress, energy, treatment space, and overall professional and personal demeanor. It is important for you to be calm and self-assured. My best advice on how to achieve this is simply to be sincere but professional at all times.

Telling the medical history in and of itself has a therapeutic effect. You need to create a safe environment for the patient that allows for the natural expression of their history. Your goal is to both get the information that you need to understand the complexity of their health and yet not put words into their mouth. The interview questions are tools to collect the data and should not get in the way or become an obstacle to seeing whom the patient really is. Do not be so concerned with the form of the interview that you lose its spirit and do not discern its content.

Medical doctor Konner (1997, p.82) noticed in his residency career,

> The patient is on the lowest rung of the hospital ladder of authority, with opinions that must be managed rather than considered. Yet ironically, it is the patient whose life is most being affected; those opinions do matter. We need to raise their opinions to the highest rung. One way to do this is through the interview.

My experience is that if the meaning of the illness can be interpreted, captured, or conveyed to the patient that true healing can begin and both you and the patient can work together to remedy the disease. The history telling, if clearly elicited, is as therapeutic as the treatment itself. Courage is needed to ask about home, life and love, loss and personal values, goals and fulfillment, illness, death and dying if they seem relevant. These larger issues are delicate and difficult to inquire about until you get into the habit of doing so. But these queries can provide the answer to the grief beneath the asthma, the anger giving rise to the neck pain, the worries creating the Stomach disorders, or the fears underpinning the back problem.

Structure the interview in an organized manner, pursuing one area of inquiry fully before moving to the next with appropriate follow-up questions as needed on thoughts that need to be pursued. The patient should feel that you are genuinely listening to them, and that you are logical, credible, and caring. The patient will get a sense of completion and trust from this style of query.

The following pointers are useful interview skills to help you better understand the patient.

INTERVIEW TIPS

1. Let the patient speak to you about his or her own life. Do not be so fixed on a certain line of questioning that you fail to hear what they are really trying to tell you. Don't second guess them or make assumptions about their experiences.

2. Allow the patient to talk about their illness. The interview should be a verbal dialogue, not a response to a questionnaire. Do not ask closed ended questions that only elicit a "yes" or "no" answer, implying that only those two answers are possible. For instance, in inquiring about elimination, do not ask, "Do you have diarrhea or constipation?" The patient may have neither, both from time to time, tendencies towards one or the other, or an alternating pattern. Ask open-ended questions, not ones that can be answered in one or two words. For example, a better way to phrase the question would be, "Could you please describe your typical bowel movements."

3. Try not to interrupt once the patient starts talking. Let the patient tell you what they have to say. Learn to listen with your whole being, eyes, ears, face, and body and resume questioning when you are sure the patient is done speaking. Because the patient perceives you as the authority figure, if you interrupt the patient, they may drop the train of thought, thinking that it is not appropriate to continue.

4. Pause for a second or two after the patient finishes speaking. Silence doesn't always mean the patient has finished an answer. The patient may be gathering thoughts to continue speaking or to enter into an area that is difficult to talk about. Even if the patient is not going to continue to say anything it gives you a chance to record observations or to gather your thoughts.

5. Allow the patient to "digress" into what appear to be stories. "Stories" about life events reveal much about the patient's attitudes toward health and illness. Healthcare practitioners who listen to stories help the patient frame health or illness in a larger context. Educator nurse Nagai-Jacobson (Nagai-Jacobsen and Burkhardt 2002, p.13) maintains, "Stories transform a two dimensional medical record into a living representation. Simply listening to someone often helps his or her healing process, avoid expensive tests, and unnecessary medications."

6. Leading questions contain values that the patient can perceive so do not ask leading questions that implicate an answer that they think you want to hear. The patient may not want to disappoint you with his or her responses or face what might be disapproval from you. As people, we try to please each other. For instance don't say, "You don't eat red meat do you?" This implies that you disapprove of eating red meat, which may or may not be the case. The patient should not be made to feel judged.

7. Patients may respond to your authority through what is called the "white coat syndrome." In this common scenario, the patient defers to you and expects you to take care of them. Through the interview establish with the patient that healing is a process that both of you will activate and explore together. They are not victims and you are not superior to them. You respect their autonomy and seek to inform it.

8. Encourage the patient to talk, argues C. Everett Koop (in Dobb 1995, p.92), former US Surgeon General. "Encouraging passivity in patients couldn't be more wrongheaded. Healthcare begins and ends with the individual who is ill and whose health is at risk."

9. If necessary, as in the case of special patients like children, teenagers, or the elderly, or in any relevant situation where there is agreement to do so, family members are interviewed at the same time, as long as confidentiality is not breached. Nagai-Jacobson (Nagai-Jacobsen and Burkhardt 2002, p.13) prompts, "Families who share life stories together can improve communication with each other, which is especially helpful

in dealing with illness. Children often lack the vocabulary to explain their feelings. The stories they tell can reveal their understanding of health and illness."

10. The choice of words patients use subjectively describes their experience better than any of our questions can. Language is an expression of the spirit. Listen to the tone of the voice, the choice of words, the Five Element sounds, the expressions and emotions conveyed in the language, the volume of the voice, and so on. According to Traditional Chinese medicine, the way in which the spirit is affected influences the flow of *Qi* and *Blood* and accordingly that affects the spirit (*Shen*) that is revealed in the language and its expression.

11. Swapping stories is a technique that practitioners have different views on. Some maintain that your experiences as a physician should never be brought up to the patient. Supposedly this ensures objectivity and the proper degree of interaction that many feel should exist between the patient and the practitioner. On the other hand, sharing stories can assist in rapport building and can make the patient feel that you do understand them and you are also human. Sharing stories can confer a degree of hope that can lead to healing. Just make sure the patient realizes that this is your story and do not let your experience take away from the patient interpreting his or her own experience. There are times when doing so is appropriate. You need to use your professional judgment.

12. Try to locate the level of discomfort of the patient. Is it the psyche (*Shen*) or the soma (Body/*Qi* and *Blood*)? In China and in many other countries where the psyche is suppressed, feelings are not attended to either for societal reasons such as loss of face, or simply because the individual is not important in that culture. In China, emotional states tend to be lumped together and somatized, and the psychosocial aspects of illness are ignored. For instance, a person's anger over their assigned occupation in China can lead to hypertension.

When only 10% of healthcare accounts for an individual's health you must look to other factors to help patients. Additionally, to help you grow your practice to be an effective, successful, and ethical healthcare provider built into community who contributes to social justice, it is necessary to know the problems of your county and even neighborhood. You need to inquire about where and a how a person lives. A very useful resource that you should consult as a practitioner embedded in community is *County Health Rankings*. At this site you can learn about the demographics of your community and the social determinants of health that may be contributing to their illness such as income level, educational level, race, ethnicity, age, and other factors that influence patient health.

PATIENT EDUCATION

Doctors should view patient education as one of their primary missions. By providing patient education related to the physical, psychological, social, and emotional issues uncovered by the patient, the etiology of much illness, especially chronic illness, can be addressed. These topics are discussed in early Chinese texts such as the *Ling Shu*, Chapter 8, and the *Nanjing*, Chapter 34, and we should read their discussions of the *Hun* (non-corporal soul), *Po* (corporal soul), *Yi* (intention), *Zhi* (intelligence), and *Zhi* (will). All of this information correlated with the Five Elements is extremely rich and as practitioners it is up to us to reflect upon those associations.

Summary

Ultimately, the interview is about establishing contact with the patient's spirit. The treatment that eventually follows is about letting the spirits do what they will so that a change is effected. The interview that you conduct is contingent upon how you see your role as a healthcare provider. Koop (in Dobb 1995, p.92) concurs stating, "We've forgotten the degree to which sound medical practice depends on skillful, sensitive communication." In my opinion it is the role of being a loving presence to the patient. Larre and Rochat de la Vallee (1990–1991, p.49) concur remarking, "Healing is not nursing or mothering. The way to care for a patient is to just be yourself and to be with him, looking into his eyes." Allow the interview to be the window to the soul of your patients. Look into their eyes.

Chapter 3

The Relationship Between the Methods of Diagnosis and Therapeutic Effectiveness

Learning Objectives

The purpose of this chapter is to set the stage for the needling process. Practitioners are reminded that needling is not independent of the diagnostic process but intimately related to it.

The Chinese methodology of intake to treatment is outlined in this chapter.

Practitioners of Oriental medicine should agree that the aim of every acupuncture treatment should be to restore balance and wholeness to the patient and thus to relieve the patient's "dis-ease." In acupuncture, the ability to achieve this end is ultimately through the utilization of the needle. Thus, excellent needle technique is extremely important in the treatment process. Yet even the best needle techniques cannot compensate for an inaccurate diagnosis or a faulty treatment plan, so these skills need to be equally developed.

The ability to arrive at a correct diagnosis is correspondingly dependent on the ability to collect the necessary diagnostic information through the classical methods of diagnosis: inspection, auscultation, olfaction, palpation, and inquiry. Then the practitioner must be able to weave the signs and symptoms of patient disharmony into a synergistic whole that portrays each individual's unique constellation of energy. In short, within classical Chinese medicine, there is an intrinsic logic that pervades the process from the first gathering of data through to therapeutic effectiveness achieved in treatment. These related steps are discussed herein, and depicted in Figure 3.1 and summarized in Table 3.1, Intake to Improvement: The Inherent Logic of the Chinese Diagnostic and Delivery Systems.

Table 3.1. Intake to Improvement: The Inherent Logic of the Chinese Diagnostic and Delivery Systems

Goal	The Health of the Patient
Step 1	Perform the methods of diagnosis
Step 2	Organize the data into a diagnostic framework
Step 3	Arrive at a diagnosis
Step 4	Formulate a treatment principle
Step 5	Select the appropriate treatment modality
Step 6	Select the points to be needled Provide the rationale for each point's use and determine the method of needling
Step 7	Administer treatment
Step 8	Evaluate therapeutic effectiveness
Step 9	Continually reassess and return to Step 1

Step 1

Collect the data necessary to arrive at a diagnosis through inspection, auscultation, olfaction, palpation, and inquiry. Together, these methods, organized around the senses and the intellect, allow the practitioner to gather the fullest possible range of data about the patient.

Step 2

Assess the situation, that is, organize the data into the appropriate and/or preferred diagnostic framework. Each framework, like a lens, helps the practitioner to view the person from a unique and clear perspective. Preferred paradigms are often a function of how much exposure the practitioner has had to them. Their effectiveness is directly linked to the ability of that paradigm to contribute to seeing the "picture" of the patient. Pictures of reality are ways of viewing the world. They can range from photographic preciseness, to impressionistic imagery, to the energetic expression of modern art. Each diagnostic paradigm, like a picture, is a vision, no better and no worse than the other, as long as it contributes to organizing the experience of the patient. Acupuncture paradigms, the "pictures," used to organize the expression of the patient, include the following:

- *Yin/Yang*

- *Qi* and *Blood*

- Three Treasures (*Qi, Jing, Shen*)

- Four Levels (*Wei, Qi, Ying, Xue*)

- Five elements (Wood, Fire, Earth, Metal, Water)

- Six divisions (*Taiyang, Shaoyang, Yangming, Taiyin, Shaoyin, Jueyin*)

- *Zang-fu* organs

- Essential substances (*Qi, Blood, Jin-ye, Jing, Shen, Marrow*)

- Eight principles (internal–external, excess–deficient, *Yin–Yang*, hot–cold)

- Extraordinary vessels

- *Jing luo* (meridian therapy)

- *Luo* vessels

- *San Jiao*

- Exogenous pathogens of wind, cold, damp, dryness, heat, and summer heat

- Endogenous pathogens, the emotions of anger, joy, fear, fright, grief, worry, and sadness

- Miscellaneous pathogens, that is, neither exogenous nor endogenous pathogens. They include factors such as diet, exercise, trauma, scars, radiation, and so on

- Secondary pathological products of stagnant *Blood*, Damp-phlegm

- Energetic layers of skin, muscle, meridian, blood, organ, and bone

- Western medical model and its etiological factors

- Japanese systems

- Palpatory findings

- Heaven-Man-Earth

- Others you may know

In order to arrive at a diagnosis, the practitioner must artistically and carefully weave the data from the physical exam with the voluminous information revealed in the interview. Thus, a coherent and accurate assessment can be achieved. The interview process described in Chapter 2 is the heart of the clinical encounter.

Step 3

Identify the problem, that is, arrive at a diagnostic statement. Like a hypothesis, the diagnostic statement is an educated guess, a tentative assumption based on facts, about what is going on with the person. It should be an artful, clear, simple statement. It is a summary of the patient's present as it relates to his or her past, for example, Liver *Blood* deficiency that has become Liver *Qi* stagnation. The fact that a diagnosis is not final, just as no hypothesis is final until it has been verified, is an important guiding principle in treatment. The practitioner must evaluate this hypothesis and modify it every time the patient is seen.

Step 4

Formulate a treatment principle, that is, a therapeutic plan directly related to the diagnosis. For example, a diagnostic statement of "Spleen *Qi* deficiency" has a treatment plan of "Tonify the *Qi* of the Spleen."

Step 5

Select the appropriate treatment modalities that have known clinical effectiveness in treating the diagnosed condition. The most common modalities include, but are not limited to the following:

- Acupuncture and its microsystems, such as auricular therapy, scalp acupuncture, hand acupuncture, or others

- Moxibustion

- Cupping

- Plum blossom needle therapy

- *Gwa Sha*

- Herbal medicine

- *Tuina*

- Massage

- Nutritional therapy

- Exercise/breathing therapy

- Lifestyle changes

Step 6

If acupuncture is used, select the points to be needled. Provide the rationale for each point's use and determine the method of needling, that is, tonification or dispersion. For example, tonify BL 18 (*Ganshu*), *Back Shu* point of the Liver to nourish the Liver *Blood*. Tonify LR 4 (*Zhongfeng*), the metal point on the wood meridian, to move the Liver *Qi* stagnation because metal controls wood.

Step 7

Administer treatment. Verify that there is a correlation between the treatment plan and what is actually done. That is, if the strategy is to tonify, make sure that the needle technique is indeed a tonification technique.

Step 8

Evaluate therapeutic effectiveness after administering each treatment.

Step 9

Continually reassess other active problems in subsequent visits.

Although the steps detailed here are expressed linearly, they are actually cyclically related to each other. Each step leads to and prompts the next one, influencing it so the circle of wholeness and health is achieved. The interrelated steps bend into circles, all organized around the goal of treatment, which is to restore the patient to balance. Health is a reflection of that balance.

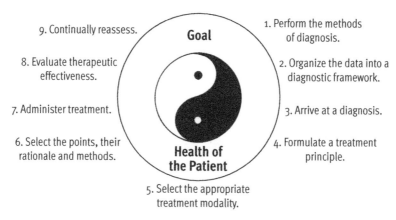

Figure 3.1: Intake to Improvement: The Inherent Logic of the Chinese Diagnostic and Delivery Systems

This is the exquisite logic of Oriental medicine that must guide the practitioner in treatment. If the results are not satisfactory, the practitioner is encouraged to look back at all of these steps to see if:

- They are all being performed to the best of one's ability

- They are mutually related to each other

- The therapeutic effect is actually being achieved. For instance, is a tonification or a dispersion technique being applied to the needle?

The intent of this book is neither on how to perform the methods of diagnosis nor on what the data collected from these procedures means. Neither is it to explain how to plug that information into established diagnostic frameworks that dictate diagnoses and suggest treatment principles. Rather, the theme of this book is how to select treatment modalities from the acupuncture techniques that have proven clinically effective in the treatment of select foundational disease patterns. Still, it is imperative to remind practitioners that the diagnostic process is full of intricacies that must be cultivated so that the best interests of their patients are served.

Practitioners also need to be mindful that the success of any treatment is not simply a function of the steps listed above, although these are critical variables. Experienced practitioners are aware that the practitioner–patient relationship is the context within which the delivery of healthcare is provided. This relationship, according to classical Chinese medicine, is not operating at its most effective level when it is only a mechanical process of gathering information and administering a treatment. A caring atmosphere of concern and confidentiality, mutual respect and rapport, professionalism and attention to the patient's presence is meaningful to bringing the patient back to health and balance. The practitioner's belief in the medicine and in her or his own abilities are empowering and will create a mindset and ambiance whereby the patient receives the best care the practitioner has to give.

Summary

If the *Neijing* (The Yellow Emperor's Classic) is correct, that healing represents a change and moves the patient's spirit, then there are many modalities to effect that change. Obviously, acupuncture is a powerful healing tool and the allied Chinese medical arts are effective as both independent and supplementary modalities. But sometimes such change can be elicited from touch, palpation, talk, laughter, and even silence, in short, from the ability of the practitioner to engage the patient's spirit. The highest level of the practice of healing then is not exclusively the logical aspects of diagnosis and treatment but the ability of one human spirit to make meaningful contact with another. As such, healing is a sacred and noble endeavor. Case 1 provides an example of the complexity of the Chinese diagnostic and delivery systems.

CASE 1: TREATING THE FOUNDATION: INSOMNIA AND PULSES AT THE ADAPTIVE LEVEL

The reading of emotions through the pulse had never been my focus until the following case. True, I had always noticed a strong correlation between grief and Lung pulses as well as between fear and Kidney pulses. Of course, a particularly wiry pulse seemed to have aggravation, irritability, or anger associated with it. The case presented herein however was one of the most difficult I ever treated. There were many reasons for this, but the lack of patient compliance was the major problem. It also illustrates how to interpret very deep pulses as manifestations of emotions that have been habituated to.

Sleep disorders are America's most frequent, deadliest, and costliest malady. A particular strength of the Chinese medical paradigm is that it gives an internal perspective on why insomnia develops. It is this precise differentiation that assists the practitioner in successful treatment. However, it is important to keep in mind that the emotions that accompany insomnia often make it difficult to treat. The patients are tired, frequently irritable, and sometimes desperate during their waking hours without having had rest.

The patient in this case was a fifty-seven-year-old female who had developed a sleeping disorder about four months previously. Her sleep pattern was characterized by an intense desire to go to bed early only to wake up three to five times during the night. She was clearly frantic.

Poor memory, lassitude, daytime drowsiness, dizziness, poor appetite, being easily frightened, shortness of breath, pallor, dry skin, and a stifling sensation in the chest also characterized her variety of sleeplessness. In addition, one of her arms twitched involuntarily. The pulse was deep and thready with an irregularity. The tongue, which was slightly purple with a red tip and almost no coat, was slightly deviated, wet, and quivery. Her insomnia was primarily of a deficient origin. In particular it was caused by a lack of the essential substances of *Qi* and *Blood* that were failing to anchor the spirit *(Shen)*, thus resulting in wakefulness.

One year previously she had experienced an unidentified illness in which the symptoms were fever, swollen glands, and lethargy. She had worked extremely hard for a number of years "because it was necessary" and at that time her energy was "super." It had been a difficult time emotionally yet, "That is just the way it was," she reported. She clearly did not want to elaborate. About three years before seeing me she became noticeably colder, particularly in the evening. She lives in a very cold house in the mountains with no source of heat.

Firstly, I ascertained that her spirit *(Shen)* needed to be treated, quieted, and calmed so that it would descend and become anchored in the material substrates of *Qi* and *Blood*. The problem was that *Qi* and *Blood* were inadequate and hence could not fulfill this function. The treatment strategy was a delicate balancing act of bringing the energy down from the head and rooting it, while simultaneously securing it by building *Qi* and *Blood*. To bring down the energy was rather easy and she was able to sleep once treatments began. But to hold it there was difficult and lasted only temporarily due to the *Qi* and *Blood* deficiency that takes time to build. The results were not permanent but confirmatory of the diagnosis.

The patient demanded immediate and long-lasting results. Every successful step in treatment was a morsel, a promise of what was to come, and the patient voraciously clamored for more. In addition, the patient did things that I thought could be exacerbating her condition. These activities included inversion therapy (hanging upside down), hypnosis, and hot baths before bed, sleeping on a magnetic bed, cranial-sacral therapy, elixir energy drinks, sleeping pills, and bizarre "blood purification" techniques. Because the patient moved from therapy to therapy, it was impossible to determine the effects of the therapies, positive or negative, if there were any at all, but overall they seemed to be contributing to her insomnia.

The patient responded very well to acupuncture and moderately well to Chinese herbs. She always slept very well after a treatment. This pattern continued to improve for several months, but the results would only last for a few days at a time. More frequent visits were indicated, but were limited because the patient lived quite a distance away and was very conservative with her money.

After two months of sporadic treatment, the pulse, which had been so thin, but more importantly too deep, began to rise. There was a palpable Kidney pulse and the pulse in general was rising to the level appropriate for that time of year. At this point, I requested that the patient undergo some Western medical tests to refine the diagnosis. Even though significant improvement had been made in a short time with very little treatment, the patient was more dissatisfied and difficult to work with than ever. Her dalliance with other therapies made it hard for me to achieve stability in her case. There were other factors, such as hysteria, personal onslaughts on me as to why she could not sleep better, and the need to travel to my office that complicated the case. Also, she refused to see a Western physician because she was sure a medical condition would be discovered that her insurance company would not cover. All of this set up the dynamics for a therapeutic relationship that reached an impasse. This case presents several different lessons, not the least of which is to do the best we can and not become too attached to the outcome which ultimately is not controlled by the practitioner.

Looking at the pathology, it was obvious that this patient's difficulties, supported by numerous signs and symptoms, centered around the Heart, its willingness to give, to receive, to laugh, to rest, and to harmonize with the social world. The deep weak pulses indicated that her problem was related to the internal organs and to the *Yin* organs in particular. It was a chronic problem that had been adapted to. As the recuperative, foundational energy of the body was tapped and strengthened through needling, the pulse became stronger and higher. The emotions, even if in the form of complaints, began to surface, to be expressed, instead of being buried at the deep, hidden, adaptive level of the pulse. The deepest level of human energy, the *Shen* or spirit, had been reached, nourished, and secured, to now allow the foundational energy of *Qi* and *Blood* to be built. Now the patient needed to attend to her feelings and redirect them harmoniously to the world.

Summary

Take the time before rushing to treatment to be clear of your goal, the health of the patient, and to logically link your processes from intake to assessment. Treating the foundation is the key to long-lasting results.

Chapter 4

Thoughts on Needling Within the Clinical Encounter

Learning Objectives

This chapter teaches the basis of all needling—practitioner awareness of the spirit of the needle—and how that needle connects to the spirit (*Shen*) of the patient.

The *Neijing* (*The Yellow Emperor's Classic*), the oldest Chinese medical text, states (as quoted in Larre and Rochat de Valle 1990–1991, p.48), "The key to acupuncture lies in regulating the mind." This statement has been explained by modern practitioners of Chinese medicine in China to mean that the accomplished acupuncturist must center their mind on the needle. Another dramatic quote from the same sources admonishes, "Needling is like looking at a deep abyss; take care not to fall… Your hand must be like a hand grasping a tiger. One desires a kind of firm strength."

The *Neijing*, according to the Chinese doctors I studied with, says,

> When caring for a patient concentrate on the situation without being distracted by the circumstances, as if standing on the brink of a gorge and not wanting to fall in. When you grasp the needle do so with great care, firm strength and caution of the peril, as if holding a tiger's tail; one wrong move and great harm could befall.

Although ancient as well as modern practitioners recognize the legal implications of poor needle execution, these striking statements refer more to the seriousness and profundity of misusing a needle in another person's body. Other quotes reinforce these concepts of wielding a needle and the importance of having a clear mind.

> Know that you are the edge of the mystery of life. Walk on the edge of the abyss without fear but have caution and circumspection not to fall. As a practitioner you must be deeply anchored and assured in your life. Yet the communication with the exterior passes through your orifices and your hand, which is holding the needle like a hand trying to hold a tiger. The tiger is the image of vital power. (As quoted in Larre and Rochat de Valle 1990–1991, p.48)

Anything healthcare practitioners do in their own lives to develop consciousness, attentiveness, and awareness will support their work as acupuncturists with intent. Whether it is gardening, calligraphy, painting, or housework, or an infinite number of other tasks in which mindfulness is required, the goal is to bring full presence and attentiveness to the activity at hand. In the case of needling, the practitioner must possess the appropriate consciousness, for as the *Ode to the Explanation of Mysteries* notes (quoted in Dale 1994, p.2), "If you should want to treat illness, there is nothing so good as the needle."

Health is not simply a product of homeostasis initiated by inserting a needle. It is a positive vision of a person ample in *Qi* and *Blood*, glowing with the vitality of the life force, whose materiality, spirit, and emotions are products of the Upright *Qi* of the body. It is the responsibility of practitioners to possess this mindfulness, to visualize this possibility of human existence, every time a patient is treated. Acupuncture is not simply the insertion of a needle into the body that then automatically corrects its imbalances. The classics (quoted in Dale 1994, p.167) reinforce this fact when they state, "The unskilled physician grasps only the form when he uses the techniques of acupuncture. The superior physician understands the spirit." We must safeguard the gift of life with the instrument of the needle. This ancient understanding of the treatment of disease portrays human life as the integration of physical, emotional, and spiritual energies. If the practitioner only adopts a material point of view when treating the human body, by definition they will not succeed.

If the patient's illness has not been corrected, there are many variables that need to be reviewed. For example, the practitioner must know whether to tonify or to disperse and then make sure that the needle technique actually executed was indeed a tonification or a dispersion technique. Even with all this, if the treatment is too materialistically oriented, too mechanistic, only the physical form, not the totality of the person's essence will have been grasped. Still, if the practitioner does not know how to manipulate the needle, the highest level of understanding of theory and the ability to utilize theory and arrive at a diagnosis that captures the essence of the person is useless.

According to the Chinese doctors I studied with in Beijing, the *Neijing* postulates, "As if perched above a fathomless abyss with one hand grasping a tiger [when holding the needle] the spirit must not be distracted by anything." To hold the needle as if holding the tiger's tail is a dangerous, magical, and powerful act. The willingness to accept this danger and opportunity is as necessary to treatment as it is to living. I urge all practitioners to have the fearful respect to hold the tiger's tail.

Summary

Acupuncturists must cultivate this knowledge to adjust the flow of energy before they have the privilege of inserting a needle into the human body. These adages prompt reflection.

Chapter 5

The Stages of Needling

Learning Objectives

The goal of this chapter is to illustrate the distinct steps involved from the insertion to the withdrawal of a needle. If the practitioner can visualize these stages, and then practices them, needling should be painless and effective.

Although the well-executed needle may seem to melt into the body through a good Chinese needle technique, or sink into the skin painlessly with a solid Japanese style, there are actually several integral steps to proficient needling that are not always apparent to the untrained eye because of the finesse of the skilled practitioner. These phases are delineated herein. The practitioner is encouraged to practice these steps on inanimate objects such as cotton balls tied together before using on a patient.

THE SIX STAGES OF NEEDLING
1. Insertion: painless and sterile

Insertion involves getting the needle into the skin in a sterile and painless manner. The epidermis is the outermost layer of the skin. It has five sub-layers. The outermost layer is made up of 10–30 layers of continuously shedding cells. Beneath the epidermis is the dermis, which has two sub-layers, and where the free nerve endings are located. Sterile means that the shaft of the needle is not compromised by being touched with the bare hand.

When using Chinese needles, the classics prescribe, assuming one is right-handed (Bensky and O'Connor 1981, p.407), "The left hand is heavy and presses hard (on the point). This causes the *Qi* to disperse. The right hand is light for entry and exit. In this way there is no pain." Here, the acupuncturist is instructed in a two-handed needle technique where the point to be needled is pressed with one hand to stimulate the *Qi* of the channels and separate free nerve endings while the needle is inserted by the dominant hand with a thrust. When using an insertion tube with either a Chinese or Japanese needle, painless insertion can be achieved by firmly hitting the handle of the needle with the pad of the index finger as opposed to lightly tapping the head repeatedly.

Common errors that acupuncturists who use needles with tubes often make, and that cause unnecessary pain to the patient, include the following:

1. Failing to disengage or detach the needle from the tube before attempting to tap it in.

2. Letting the needle tip sit too long on the skin before insertion. This causes pain.

3. Pushing the needle in inadvertently as it rests on the skin.

Painless and sterile insertions are necessary for good needle technique and patient health.

2. Going to the level of the *Qi*

Once the needle has been inserted without pain and in a sterile manner, it must now be inserted to the level of the *Qi*, that is, where the *Qi* resides. It is common knowledge that each point has a particular insertion depth that is determined by anatomical landmarks and meridian energetics. Underlying anatomical structures such as vital organs, tendons, ligaments, major blood vessels, nerves, bone foramina, and so on, as well as individual variations in the patient's body size, sex, age, constitution, excesses, deficiencies, and the nature of the illness, dictate where the *Qi* will most likely be encountered. The practitioner's experience and treatment plan are also factors. No therapeutic result can be anticipated if the needle is not inserted to the level where the vital energy resides.

3. Getting the *Qi*

After the needle has been inserted to the level of the *Qi*, the *Qi* must now be contacted and engaged. Getting the *Qi* is half of the battle. This is the essence of needling. Without getting the *Qi*, the treatment plan cannot proceed; that is, no subsequent tonification or dispersion can be initiated if the *Qi* has not been contacted.

Techniques to getting the *Qi* are analogous to fishing. Teasing the energy in the body to the needle is like attracting a fish to the bait. The arrival of *Qi* feels like a fish taking the line. Typically, a feeling of tightness or fullness signifies the arrival of *Qi* of a needle in rubber, or the fish taking the bait. Common methods for getting the *Qi* include but are not limited to the following, which are discussed herein and summarized in Table 5.1, Techniques for Getting the *Qi*.

Lift and thrust

Perpendicularly lift and thrust the needle but without too much force or the tissues may become damaged. This action coaxes the *Qi* to the needle on a vertical axis.

Twirl

Continuously rotate the needle back and forth, with small rotations in search of the *Qi* on the horizontal axis. Never rotate the needle only in one direction as this action entwines the tissues and can cause pain.

Tremble

In a movement termed the "trembling technique," use a simultaneous lift and thrust method with the twirling technique to attract the *Qi* to the point. This is my preferred technique.

Retain the needle and wait for the *Qi* to arrive

Many practitioners do this but this method is overall ineffectual unless while waiting the following strategies are employed.

PRESS ALONG THE MERIDIAN, ALSO CALLED A FOLLOWING TECHNIQUE

With the needle in place, press along the course of the meridian both above and below the needle to stimulate the vital Qi, which may be weak and lead the Qi to the needle.

PLUCK

Pluck the handle of the needle to cause a vibration along the length of the needle into the meridian. This method will smooth the Qi along the channel in the event of any stagnation that is contributing to the slow arrival of the Qi.

SHAKE

Shake the needle to strengthen the needle's presence, assist in the arrival of Qi, and displace any perverse pathogen.

SCRAPE

Scrape the fingernail along the spiral head of a Chinese needle in an upward direction to bring the Qi to the point.

ROTATE AND RELEASE

Use a "flying needle" technique. This consists of rotating the needle in one direction until resistance is encountered and then suddenly releasing the needle. Repeat this movement three times. This method propagates and prolongs the needling sensation.

NEEDLE A POINT NEARBY

Needle a point nearby and along the course of the meridian to summon the Qi to the point.

APPLY MOXA

Apply moxa to the affected area to promote the circulation of Qi to the point.

Of course, in addition to manipulation methods, there are other factors that influence the arrival of Qi to a point. Some of the most important are correct point location, angle and depth of insertion, the age and constitution of the person, and the skill of the practitioner.

Table 5.1. Techniques for Getting the *Qi*

1.	Lift and thrust
2.	Twirl
3.	Tremble: this is a simultaneous lift and thrust and twirl
4.	Retain and wait and choose one of the following: • Press along the course of the meridian • Pluck the handle • Shake the needle • Scrape the handle • Rotate and release • Needle a point nearby • Apply moxa

4. Manipulating the *Qi*

After the *Qi* arrives (called *Da Qi*), something must be done with it. The engaged *Qi* must be manipulated to achieve the therapeutic purpose of either strengthening and invigorating (tonifying) or dispersing (sedating, draining, or breaking up) the energy. My Chinese teachers continue to reiterate that while half of the battle is getting the *Qi*, the other half is what is done with it. Without attention to both these aspects of needle technique, the aim of the treatment will not be accomplished.

The Chinese treat most diseases with needle retention. The needle retention time strengthens and deepens the action of the technique. Conventional needle retention times for tonification and dispersion have been established, but in the final analysis, needles only have to be retained until the practitioner is sure that the goal of the treatment has been reached.

There are other indications of therapeutic effectiveness that are more reliable than time, predominantly the needle technique itself. A change in the patient's pulse or demeanor, feeling the stimulus or a reaction to the stimulus, and also the skin's color can indicate that it is time to remove the needle.

Table 5.2, Concepts of Tonification and Dispersion: Getting the *Qi* and Manipulating the Reaction, summarizes some of the most common methods of tonifying and dispersing found in the literature and in clinical practice. Other techniques can be found in books about the treatment of disease as well as in journal articles. It is to the advantage of the patient that the practitioner be cognizant and proficient with as many techniques as possible so that various patient presentations can be treated.

Table 5.2. Concepts of Tonification and Dispersion:
Getting the *Qi* and Manipulating the Reaction

Variables	Tonification	Dispersion
Size of needles	Use thin needles	Use thick needles
Number of needles	Needle fewer points	Needle more points
Body type	For thin constitutional types	For heavier constitutional types
Condition	For chronic conditions	For acute conditions
When	Needle when the channel is weak (see channel's horary cycle time)	Needle when the channel is full (see channel's horary cycle time)
Moon	Needle at the new moon as the energy of the universe is increasing and supplementing	Needle at the full moon when the energy of the universe is full and the energy needs to be drained
Depth	• Needle superficially • Press the point heavily with the hand and insert the needle deeply	• Needle deeply • Insert shallowly
Type of needles	Use gold or copper needles (yellow metals, which are *Yang*) to strengthen	Use silver needles (white metals, which are *Yin*) to cool
Other modalities	Use moxa, needles, exercise, diet, *Qi Gong*, rest, herbs	Use needles as the primary treatment modality
Types of points	Choose points that are tonification points or have tonifying energetics	Choose points that are dispersion points or have dispersion energetics

Direction and action relative to the meridian	• Insert the needle in the direction of the meridian flow • For points of the Three Hand *Yang* and Three Foot *Yin* turn the needle clockwise • For points of the Three Hand *Yin* and Three Foot *Yang* turn the needle counter-clockwise	• Insert the needle in the opposite direction of the meridian flow • For points of the Three Hand *Yang* and Three Foot *Yin* turn the needle counter-clockwise • For points of the Three Hand *Yin* and Three Foot *Yang* turn the needle clockwise
Lift/Thrust	Lift the needle slowly and gently, thrust heavily and rapidly	Lift the needle forcibly and rapidly, thrust gently and slowly
Amplitude and speed	Turn the needle with small amplitude (rotation) and slow speed	Turn the needle with large amplitude (rotation) and fast speed
Sensation	Achieve no or a mild needling sensation	Achieve a strong needling sensation
Time	Retain needles from 3–20 minutes. Some sources say tonification should be longer than dispersion	Retain needles from 20 minutes to 1 hour. Some sources say dispersion should be shorter than tonification
Insertion and withdrawal	• Insert the needle slowly and withdraw quickly • Insert on the inhale, withdraw on exhale • Insert on the exhale, withdraw on inhale	• Insert the needle quickly and withdraw slowly • Insert on the exhale, withdraw on inhale • Insert on the inhale, withdraw on exhale
Site	Apply pressure by closing the hole with a clean, dry cotton ball immediately after taking the needle out	Enlarge the hole upon withdrawal by shaking the needle and leave the hole open
Direction	One large clockwise turn followed by three small counter-clockwise turns	Three small counter-clockwise turns followed by one large clockwise turn
Type of person	Shallow depth for more sensitive patients	Deep and strong for less sensitive patients
Condition	Deficiency	Excess

(continued)

Variables	Tonification	Dispersion
Frequency	Once or intermittently, i.e., manipulate slightly for a few seconds, rest, and repeat	Vigorously or continuously until symptoms are relieved from several minutes to several hours as in the case of anesthesia
Moxibustion	Apply more	Apply less

Notes

- Tonification and dispersion are always relative.
- There are conflicting different points of view on some of the methods.

REACTION
5. Withdrawal

Needles should be carefully and gently removed. Force should never be used to disengage a needle from a point. If a needle appears to be stuck, it may have been inserted too forcefully or manipulated too vigorously and in the future the practitioner should be more careful. If the practitioner does experience such a situation when withdrawing the needle the following approaches can be tried:

1. Gently massage around another point close by to attract the *Qi* from the stuck needle.

2. Needle another point in close proximity for similar reasons.

3. If the needle seems to be entwined in the tissue, try to turn it slowly in the opposite direction to disengage it.

6. Dealing with the site

The final stage of needling, following withdrawal of the needle, concerns the needle site. Table 5.2 also summarizes commonly accepted notions of what to do with the puncture site after needling (that is, close the hole for tonification or leave it open for dispersion). In the event of bleeding or ecchymosis, the practitioner, regardless of tonification or dispersion technique, should absorb the blood with a sterile cotton ball and apply pressure to the bruised or tender area. Figure 5.1, The Six Stages of Needling, shows the stages of needling in graphic form.

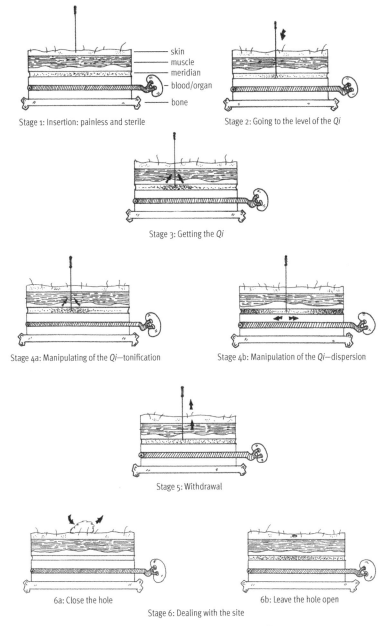

Figure 5.1: The Six Stages of Needling

Summary

Acupuncture is the insertion of needles into the human body for the purposed of adjusting the energy of the body. Acupuncture cannot be done if the needle cannot enter the body sterilely and painlessly, if the *Qi* is not contacted, or if the *Qi* is not manipulated to effect a change. Needling is not difficult but it is a conscious, thoughtful act. Visualize and practice needling in order to treat your patients effectively.

Chapter 6

What Is an Acupuncture Point?

Learning Objectives

In this chapter the reader can explore the physiological parameters of bodily acupuncture points that aid in assisting the understanding of the actions of each point.

The classics (in Larre and Rochat de Vallee 1990–1991) remind us that the aim of the five branches of Oriental healing therapy is to establish a connection between the patient and the practitioner, and to effect a change in the body. Whether that change is through acupuncture, herbs, massage, nutrition, or exercise/breathing therapy we seek to change pathological energy and rectify it. In acupuncture, where the tool for this connection is the needle, three factors—correct needle technique, coupled with precise point location, and astute point selection—are prerequisite to achieving the desired therapeutic result of effecting a change.

The energetics or functions of the points are numerous and essentially correspond to the physiological functions of the body. They are not identical to the indications of the points, which are disease conditions the person may have such as a headache. The indications flow from the point energetics. The clinical experience of Chinese medicine suggests that the points are capable of correcting the physiological deficiencies that humans are prone to unless the vital *Qi* is so diminished or deranged that the imbalance cannot be redressed.

Because of the proliferation of point indications that have been developed over the years, the beginning student or novice practitioner of Oriental medicine often becomes lost in remembering those indications and more importantly why those points possess those indications. They struggle to see some rhyme or reason as to why each point possesses the indications they had to routinely memorize. But there are reasons as to why a point does what it does. This is what I call the classical energetics of the points.

If one thing can be said about Oriental medicine, apart from its effectiveness as shown throughout the centuries, it is that it is an inherently logical medicine. That is not to say that there are not competing paradigms within its vast body of experience for there are. These apparent inconsistencies are actually a source of strength to the system because of the options they present. However, the Chinese medical system is logical in the sense that pathology, i.e. indications, can be predicted if physiology is understood. Point energetics are a product of the classical, physiological roles those points play in the organism.

The role of points in the human body can be viewed from a variety of perspectives. The Chinese remind us that in discussing the identity of acupuncture points, both the anatomic and physiologic aspects of the points need to be considered. That is, where the point is located anatomically, and what the point does physiologically, are contributing factors to understanding the energetics of points. The way I like to think about the points, which concurs with this Chinese assessment, is that where a point "lives," that is its anatomical location, and what a point does, that is its physiological function, are akin to a "job description" that contributes to its unique identity.

A survey of the acupuncture literature offers further insight into the question, "What is a point?" Etymologically, the word for point, *Xue*, denotes a cave or hole. This translation suggests how the Chinese viewed this site. The word also evokes the notion that demons, especially wind demons, could live in these holes, either in nature or in the body. Over time, this hole, according to Unschuld (1985), came to connote a place where *Qi* was able to penetrate into the body as well as flow out. The Chinese character for "hole" was combined with the character for "passage, transport, and *Qi*" so that the point came to be perceived as a route to the interior or the exterior. As such, the points were channels of communication between the external and internal environments. Pathogens could enter the body here. The *Spiritual Axis*, according to Bensky and O'Connor (1981, p.401), claimed, "Points are places where the *Qi* roams in and out."

Classically, the points were viewed as anatomical locations on the body where the *Qi* and *Blood* could be accessed. Points were seen as sites where the *Qi* of the *Zang-fu* organs and channels is transported to the body surface. Because there are relative excesses and deficiencies in the body, the points were considered as places where these imbalances could be approached and changed. When the human body is affected by disease, we can treat the patient by puncturing points on the surface of the body to regulate the *Qi* and *Blood* of the channels. The image of the point as a hole or a gate that allows the entry and exit of *Qi* provides a living, functional image of the point as an active physiological nexus embedded within an anatomical location. So, for example, if we want to bring energy to the point, we "tonify" it; if we want to take energy away from an area through the point, we "disperse" or sedate it. The various ways of accomplishing these two basic movements of energy are listed in Table 5.2, found in Chapter 5.

There are further anatomical analogies that support the model of a point as a working physiological location that can reflect the point's job description. Historically, one definition of points included areas that had different consistencies, colorations, or were more moist or dry than surrounding areas (Bensky and O'Connor 1981). This description points to the importance of cultivating perception through inspection and palpation by the practitioner, thus assisting not only in point location but diagnosis as well. Other findings that support the contention that points reflect "physiology gone wrong" can be found in Table 6.1, Signs of Point Pathology Derived from the Five Methods of Diagnosis.

The *Neijing* posits a maxim that most acupuncturists are well aware of, that is, where there is a painful spot, there is an acupuncture point. The significance of this statement is that pain or discomfort from either excess or deficiency represents pathology in the body. Sometimes such pain is overt, that is, the patient is aware of it and articulates it either as a major complaint or as part of their internal landscape. Other times though, pain is below the threshold of consciousness and can only be significantly evoked and grappled with when the body is palpated.

Table 6.1. Signs of Point Pathology Derived from the Five Methods of Diagnosis

Inspection	Auscultation	Olfaction	Palpation	Inquiry
rashes	gurgling	Five	Pain:	All of the
moles	fluid	Element	referred	pathology
warts	accumulation	smells:	sharp	related to
petechiae	sounds	scorched	fixed	the Five
depressions	inhalations	fragrant	stabbing	Preliminaries
asymmetries	exhalations	rotten	boring	and the Ten
boils	sounds, sighs,	putrid	dull	Questions
lumps	and so on	rancid	awareness	
lesions			burning	
varicosities			hot	
scars			deep	
bruises			superficial	
swellings			gummy	
edema			knots	
puffiness			pulsations	
bloating			visible	
redness			tension	
bone growths			mushiness	
dryness			softness	
wetness			lack of tone	
inversions			hard like a	
eversions			rock	
knots			cold	
hair presence			dry	
hair absence			wet	
buffalo hump				
fat (overweight)				
leanness				
gauntness				
leathery				
withered				
prolapses				
growths				
sternocostal				
angle				
pulsations				
depth of				
breathing				
posture				
muscle bands				
flushing				
colorations				
birthmarks				

We must remember that one of the methods of traditional diagnosis is palpation. Because of time constraints in a student clinic setting, and even in major hospitals in China, palpation has in my opinion become an almost lost art. While it is not the purpose of this book to summarize all of the advantages of palpation that elevate it to the most subtle and sublime of diagnostic arts, it is still important to point out that precise point location can often be ascertained through inspection and palpation of suspect areas. For more information on palpation see my book, *The Art of Palpatory Diagnosis*, devoted entirely to the subject of palpation.

Acupuncture, defined as the needling of points on the human body for the purpose of adjusting the flow of energy in the body, is a means of affecting what goes on inside the body because it influences the activity of the substances moving through the meridians. As Ted Kaptchuk (1983) so eloquently and aptly summarized, stimulating points can reduce what is excessive, increase what is deficient, warm what is cold, cool what is hot, circulate what is stagnant, move what is congealed, stabilize what is reckless, raise what is falling, and lower what is rising.

In short, considering the Chinese outlook, a point can be viewed as an anatomical location through which exogenous pathogens can enter and be dispersed or through which the physiological function of the human body can be regulated and stimulated. See Figure 6.1, What is a Point?

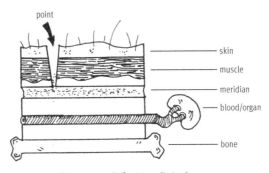

Figure 6.1: What is a Point?

Although anatomical descriptions are meaningful road maps that can denote the general area of the point, a point must be thought of as three-dimensional. Points are distinguished partly by their surface anatomical landmarks, but they also possess an underlying anatomy that can consist of organs, innervations, and vascularizations. As the *Inner Classic* states, "The twelve channels circulate deep within the muscle and cannot be seen" (Bensky and O'Connor 1981, p.111).

For different points, *Qi* resides at different depths. The functional capacity of a point is partly derived from its depth, and likewise *Qi* converges at different depths because of its anatomical location. To access the *Qi* and stimulate the appropriate point function, the correct needle technique, including the angle and depth of insertion for the particular point, and the method of needle manipulation applied to the needle, is imperative.

Seasoned practitioners know that accurate point location is not a function of mathematical divisions done on the body. Rather, because the point incarnates a living energy, a point, embedded in connective tissue could be more accurately viewed as energy in motion. Also, people vary anatomically. For instance, one may lack the tendon of the muscle palmaris longus. Another person may have six lumbar vertebrae or an attached eleventh rib. In these cases, the anatomical description of a point can only get the practitioner to the general area of the point. Palpation and inspection are unparalleled tools for the practitioner, not only in these anomalous cases but also for all correct point location.

Rubik notes (1995), Western scientists, intrigued with Oriental medicine, are not without their theories on what a point is and they have advanced a number of propositions. It is common knowledge in the scientific community that points can be electrically located, and they are considered part of the electromagnetic field of the body. It has been determined that this field is not uniformly dense. Where decreased electrical resistance and increased electrical conductivity are detected, the areas correspond to acupuncture points whose functions are deficient. Where an increase in ionic concentration is indicated by increased electrical resistance, the corresponding point function may be pathological in the Chinese sense as well, that is, there may be excess conditions such as stagnation, or presence of pathogens. These are the mechanisms whereby electropoint detectors work.

According to the Zhang–Popp hypothesis, treatment by acupuncture needling causes a disturbance in the standard wave pattern caused by a new boundary. Robert Becker and others have investigated changes in the electrical potential because of wounding such as through trauma and like that produced by needling. "Currents of injury result such that the needled region becomes a new EM [electromagnetic] field source with concomitant interference effects over the whole body" (Rubik 1995, p.45).

Using the circulatory system as the explanation for how a point works was dismissed early on because the blood and lymph flows lacked the speed with which the stimulation of an acupuncture point could affect tissues and other functions. On the other hand, nervous system involvement has been investigated and there seems to be a strong, though by no means comprehensive correlation between this regulatory system and how acupuncture works.

In 1959, researchers at the Shanghai College of Traditional Medicine (Bensky and O'Connor 1981) noted that there is a close relationship between peripheral nerves in the tissues and the acupuncture points. Of the 309 points studied, 152 points stimulated were over nerves and seventy-three were close by within 0.5 centimeters. In 1969, they noted that nerves directly supplied 323 points, superficial cutaneous nerves supplied 304, 155 were supplied by deeper nerves, and 137 had both deep and superficial involvement. From dissections and observation under microscopes, it was determined that all layers of the skin and muscle tissues at the acupuncture sites contained numerous and varied nerve endings.

Additionally, it was observed that points congregated close to nerves and consequently could be located in predictable places. The larger the peripheral nerve, especially those identifiable in gross anatomy, the more likely they were to have points distributed along them. The depth of the peripheral nerve was also an important variable. As peripheral nerves emerge from deep to superficial, points are likely to form along their nerve routes. Points could also be found where nerves penetrate the deep fascia, where a nerve emerges from a bone foramen, where a muscular branch of a peripheral nerve attaches and enters a muscle mass, and at the bifurcation point of peripheral nerves. Likewise, blood vessels were frequently seen in the vicinity of neuromuscular attachments. Points are also found at the suture lines of the skull and the sensitive points of ligaments.

Further implication of the nervous system in the action of points is found in the visceral cutaneous theory. According to this perspective, internal diseases of the organs produce pain or tenderness at certain acupuncture points or in areas of the skin known as dermatomes. This idea corresponds with Felix Mann's notion of the generalized site. This means an internal organ can become so sensitive that it can refer to a larger than normal skin area.

Although these observations represent important contributions by the modern scientific community about how acupuncture points may work, it is evident that these theories cannot explain the richness of point function that is part of the repertoire of Chinese medicine. On the other hand, the classical Chinese physicians have offered us an elegant and economical framework for organizing points devised long before a modern understanding of anatomy and physiology. They have not only helped us to comprehend and predict point indications, but they also have described mechanisms internally consistent with their theories of organ physiology, essential substances, and the etiology of disease. This, their point classification system, is discussed in Chapter 8.

Summary

When practitioners have an appreciation of anatomy and physiology as well as the Chinese idea of what a point is, the utilization of points will become more meaningful and accurate.

Chapter 7

The Importance of Standard Nomenclature of the Acupuncture Meridians and Points

Learning Objectives ———————————————

In this short chapter the importance of the World Health Organization (WHO) Standard Nomenclature for Organs and Meridians is stressed as a method for denoting meridians and points on the meridians. This nomenclature is meant to promote international cooperation and understanding especially when points are written about in professional literature. Even if a practitioner is not a professional author it is important in colleges and in private medical practice to employ WHO nomenclature as proper medical terminology through clear and consistent charting of medical records.

Acupuncture is a dynamic medicine. The theory and practice of acupuncture have been developing for more than 2500 years. It has evolved over the years through the changing Chinese dynasties and its spread to countries such as Japan and Korea (WHO 1993). Acupuncture continues to evolve in China, the United States, and many countries in the world. While the diversity and continual development of the medicine contributes to its depth, richness, and versatility, it has also led to some confusion in the modern world. This confusion stems from the fact that acupuncture developed in countries with different languages, often leading to different point names, spellings and pronunciations, different translations of the classical medical texts, and different nomenclatures for describing points and meridians.

In recent history, the practice of academic research on acupuncture has increased (WHO 1993). There are international schools of acupuncture, national licensing standards in many countries, acupuncture specialists, authors, publications, and national and international meetings dedicated to the medicine. Thus it has become increasingly important to standardize meridian and point location nomenclature for mutual understanding of the meridians and points referenced and the need for a universally accepted language of acupuncture.

Over the years various attempts had been made to standardize nomenclature but not on the global level. In an effort to reach global agreement, starting in 1982, various regional groups met for discussion and systems were devised. By 1989 a final version was created that could be used throughout the world in published literature, to alleviate confusion, and to allow for clear communication about acupuncture. The World Health Organization published the *Standard Acupuncture Nomenclature Report* followed by the second edition in 1993. It contains three parts:

1. Standardized names of the acupuncture points, including the alphanumeric code, the Chinese *Pinyin* name, and the Chinese characters.

2. Explanation of the point name, including the meaning of the characters and a brief explanation of the point.

3. Multilingual comparative list of the names of the points in English, French, Japanese, Korean, and Vietnamese. Clearly this shows that the development of standard nomenclature includes but extends beyond the important alphanumeric code, or the abbreviations of the meridian–organ systems.

The alphabetic code consists of two capital letters, for instance LU for Lung. Prior to that it was not uncommon for individual practitioners to make up their own shorthand that led to inconsistency and confusion in the written word. For instance, was L for Lung, Liver, or Large Intestine? Was Lg for Lung or Large Intestine? Was Li for Liver or Large Intestine? It makes a difference!

The alphanumeric code is easy to use. Perhaps the most awkward abbreviation is TE for Triple Energizer but note that TB, Triple Burner, the Chinese translation of *Sanjiao*, can be used.

WHO Standard Nomenclature is an extremely useful resource for students, practitioners, and researchers of Chinese medicine. Practitioners and students of Chinese medicine often underutilize the standard nomenclature, and it may not be emphasized in Chinese medical education. In addition to assisting with the issues of communication, the WHO report also emphasizes the importance of the classical names of the points, names laden with the richness of point function.

Point names over numbers may be neglected in medical education and practice. The fact that the leaders of this field gathered together to agree upon point names and meanings is a testament to the importance of preserving this ancient knowledge. It is a reminder of the insight into the energetics of the points that comes from the names given by the classical physicians.

It is essential for the community of Chinese medical students and practitioners to use this language to improve overall communication and development of the profession. As the acupuncture field continues to grow globally, this common language provides a way for clinical information and research to be discussed, recorded, and shared without ambiguity. All practitioners and students have the responsibility to be ambassadors of this medicine, and to encourage its employment. The use of standard nomenclature is a demonstration of global unity within this profession, a unity that is necessary for the continued growth and acceptance of this medicine.

To date there still appears to be hesitancy on the part of publishers to adopt a standard nomenclature and perhaps this is good in the sense that they defer to the author who should know their medicine and the professional guidelines that the community has adopted and suggest their use to their publisher. It is incumbent upon the writer to educate publishers on this standard nomenclature just as it is the duty of teachers to instruct their students as future practitioners on this acupuncture language.

As a teacher, clinician, and author with a national and international audience I agree with the WHO system and why it is used and I employ it throughout this book. I propose to the readers of this text to likewise adopt this simple, clear, and logical system in your own writing, teaching, and charting to promote professional development and international understanding.

THE WORLD HEALTH ORGANIZATION (WHO) STANDARD NOMENCLATURE FOR MERIDIANS

LU = Lung

LI = Large Intestine

SP = Spleen

ST = Stomach

HT = Heart

SI = Small Intestine

BL = Bladder

KI = Kidney

PC = Pericardium

TE or TB = Triple Energizer or Triple Burner

GB = Gall Bladder

LR = Liver

Less commonly used is the nomenclature for the Extraordinary meridians. It is as follows:

CV = Conception Vessel

GV = Governing Vessel

DV= *Dai* channel or vessel

TV= *Chong* channel or vessel

YINHV = *Yinqiao, Yin* heel vessel

YINLV= *Yinwei, Yin* linking vessel

YANGHV=*Yangqiao, Yang* heel vessel

YANGLV= *Yangwei, Yang* linking vessel

Summary

Once this simple system is used by the student early on in their acupuncture education professional habits will be established for their professional career and to support international understanding.

Chapter 8

The Point Classification System

Learning Objectives ──────────────

This chapter reacquaints the practitioner with the elegant point classification system of the acupuncture points. This paradigm makes point energetics and indications understandable and predictable, and reduces the need for memorization of how to employ a point in treatment through its rich, logical framework. Even if this chapter is only used as a review, the practitioner will strengthen their knowledge of point functions for ease and appropriateness of point selection in treatment.

Like stars in the constellations, the acupuncture points are distributed over the body along the energy pathways known as meridians. The vital, foundational energy of the body, the *Qi* and *Blood*, infuses these points. As the classics explain (Wiseman, Ellis and Zmiewski 1985), without *Qi* and *Blood* there is no place in the human body that can be living and healthy.

In answer to the question, "How many points are there?" the Chinese respond, "As many as there are painful places." However, it is important to note that these painful places are not only spots where the spontaneous firing of nerves occurs, but also locations where there is tenderness on palpation or with other mechanical stimulation such as massage by hand or with therapeutic rollers or other implements. Yet while any place in the body can exhibit pathology, there are major loci of energy that have defined locations and physiology, that is, the points of the twelve main meridians, the Conception and Governing Vessel channels, and the extraordinary points. These points make up the point classification system.

The initial classification of points begins with organizing all of the points of the human body into three major categories: the points of the fourteen channels, the Extra points, and the *Ah Shi* points. Their nature is as follows.

THE POINTS OF THE FOURTEEN CHANNELS

The points of the fourteen channels, also known as the regular points, have specific locations and actions. There are 361 points of the fourteen channels located on the twelve main meridians supplemented by the points on the Governing and Conception Vessel channels. It is not the intent of this book to discuss the unique energetics of each individual point, only major categories of points that are useful in directing thought processes about point selection. These points can be further arranged into eleven major categories that are useful in appreciating their functional roles in the body. They are discussed herein. Table 8.1, The Points of the Fourteen Channels, lists the number of points located on each channel.

Table 8.1. The Points of the Fourteen Channels

Meridian	Entry and Exit Points	Number of Points
Lung	LU 1 (*Zhongfu*) and LU 7 (*Lieque*)	11
Large Intestine	LI 4 (*Hegu*) and LI 20 (*Yingxiang*)	20
Stomach	ST 1 (*Chengqi*) and ST 42 (*Chongyang*)	45
Spleen	SP 1 (*Yinbai*) and SP 21 (*Dabao*)	21
Heart	HT 1 (*Jiquan*) and HT 9 (*Shaochong*)	9
Small Intestine	SI 1 (*Shaoze*) and SI 19 (*Tinggong*)	19
Bladder	BL 1 (*Jingming*) and BL 67 (*Zhiyin*)	67
Kidney	KI 1 (*Yongquan*) and KI 22 (*Bulang*)	27
Pericardium	PC 1 (*Tianchi*) and PC 8 (*Laogong*)	9

Triple Burner	TB 1 (*Guanchong*) and **TB 22** (*Erheliao*)	23
Gall Bladder	GB 1 (*Tongziliao*) and **GB 41** (*Zulinqi*)	44
Liver	LR 1 (*Dadun*) and LR 14 (*Qimen*)	14
Governing Vessel	GV—NONE	28
Conception Vessel	CV—NONE	24

Bold = entry and exit points that are not the 1st or last point

1. The Five *Shu* points

The Five *Shu* points, also referred to as the Five Command points, Antique points, or the Five Transporting points, are a particular collection of points on the twelve main meridians that are located between the elbow and the fingertips on the upper limbs, and between the knee and toe tips on the lower extremities. Each of the twelve main meridians has five *Shu* points. Meridians start or end externally at the *Jing* (well) points with the exception of KI 1 (*Yongquan*), which is located on the sole of the foot. Some meridians begin internally and hence internally they have no number. Regardless of the meridian, each of the Five *Shu* points has certain therapeutic properties in common that indicate how to use that point.

The energy in these Five *Shu* points is like the energy found in different bodies of water ranging from a well, to a river, to a sea, hence the concept of transporting energy. *Qi* flows in the meridians similarly to water and builds up force and depth as it flows from distal to proximal vortices that is, from the *Jing* (well) points to the *He* (sea) points. Table 8.2, The Use of the Command Points for the Amount of *Qi* They Contain, illustrates these points in terms of their analogy to a body of water, that is, the amount of *Qi* they contain. Additionally the elemental energy consigned to each point, and common clinical conditions for which each type of point can be used, can be found in that table.

Table 8.2. The Use of the Command Points for the Amount of *Qi* They Contain

Shu Point	Points on Meridian	*Yin* Meridian	*Yang* Meridian	Energy of the Point	Clinical Conditions
Jing (well)	#1 on tips of extremities (sides of nails or tips of fingers and toes)	Wood	Metal	The *Qi* of the channel starts to bubble exchanging energy to effect a change in polarity. The point stimulates the meridian as well as the tendinomuscular meridian	Sore throat, apoplexy, toothache, coma, chest fullness, mental diseases related to *Zang* organs
Ying (spring)	#2	Fire	Water	The *Qi* of the channels starts to gush; water has just started to trickle from a spring	Febrile disease
Shu (stream)	#3	Earth	Wood	The *Qi* of the channel flourishes, like a stream with stronger movement	Joint pain caused by pathogenic heat and Damp, heavy sensation of the body
Jing (river)	Not able to be consistently numbered	Metal	Fire	The *Qi* of the channel increases in abundance. There is much more flow, like the water on which boats can travel	Asthma, throat, cough disorders
He (sea)	Elbow or knee	Water	Earth	The *Qi* of the channel is the most flourishing. There are large amounts of energy going deeper	Intestinal or digestive problems, diarrhea, six *Fu* organ diseases, diseases of the Stomach and intestines

Table 8.3, Acupuncture Points that Correspond to the Five *Shu* Points, details the acupuncture point number that corresponds to the Five *Shu* points. As is obvious from the chart, if we know the number of points on a meridian, and where the meridian begins and ends, we can determine the meridian number of the *Jing* (well), *Ying* (spring), *Shu* (stream), and *Yuan* (Source) points without memorizing them.

Table 8.3. Acupuncture Points that Correspond to the Five *Shu* Points

Meridian	*Jing* (Well)	*Ying* (Spring)	*Shu* (Stream)	*Yuan* (Source)	*Jing* (River)	*He* (Sea)	*Luo*	*Xi* (Cleft)	Lower *He* (Sea)	Upper *He* (Sea)
LU	11	10	9	9	8	5	7	6	X	X
LI	1	2	3	4	5	11	6	7	ST 37	LI 9
SP	1	2	3	3	5	9	4	8	X	X
ST	45	44	43	42	41	36	40	34	X	LI 10
HT	9	8	7	7	4	3	5	6	X	X
SI	1	2	3	4	5	8	7	6	ST 39	LI 8
BL	67	66	65	64	60	40	58	63	X	X
KI	1	2	3	3	7	10	4	5	X	X
PC	9	8	7	7	5	3	6	4	X	X
TB	1	2	3	4	6	10	5	7	BL 39	X
GB	44	43	41	40	38	34	37	36	X	X
LR	1	2	3	3	4	8	5	6	X	X
GV	X	X	X	X	X	X	1	X	X	X
CV	X	X	X	X	X	X	15	X	X	X
Yinqiao	X	X	X	X	X	X	X	KI 8	X	X
Yangqiao	X	X	X	X	X	X	X	BL 59	X	X
Yinwei	X	X	X	X	X	X	X	KI 9	X	X
Yangwei	X	X	X	X	X	X	X	GB 35	X	X

X = no point

The use of the Five *Shu* points is popular, especially with classically trained practitioners, whether they are Chinese, Japanese, Korean, English, French, or Vietnamese. These are very effective points for treatment as their energetics suggest. In terms of needle technique there is sometimes a brief pricking needling sensation felt at the *Jing* (well) and *Ying* (spring) points since distal points are shallow. But good needle technique, as described in Chapter 5, at these locations, can substantially reduce discomfort. In addition, immense therapeutic advantages can generally only be achieved with these points.

The previous discussion of the Five *Shu* points has outlined how to classify these points of the human body into categories based on general energetics. These categories can help us understand the nature of a particular point, but they also have an additional property, that is, they carry an elemental energy related to the Five Elements. This energy confers upon the point its rudimentary value such as its earthy or watery nature.

The most distal *Shu* point on a *Yin* meridian is always a wood point followed by fire, earth, metal, and water in the order of the Five Elements. For instance, on the Lung meridian, LU 11 (*Shaoshang*), the *Jing* (well) point and the most distal *Shu* point, is the wood point. LU 10 (*Yuji*), the *Ying* (spring) point, is the fire point; LU 9 (*Taiyuan*), the *Shu* (stream) point, is the earth point. LU 8 (*Qingqu*), the *Jing* (river) point, is the metal point and finally, LU 5 (*Chize*), the *He* (sea) point, is the water point.

On a *Yang* meridian, the most distal *Shu* point is always a metal point. Correspondingly, the rest of the distal *Shu* points have water, wood, fire, and earth energy assigned to them in that order. For instance, the *Shu* points of the Large Intestine meridian are LI 1 (*Shangyang*), *Jing* (well) point; LI 2 (*Erjian*), *Ying* (spring) point; LI 3 (*Sanjian*), *Shu*(stream) point; LI 5 (*Yangxi*), *Jing* (river) point; and LI 11 (*Quchi*), the *He* (sea) point. These *Shu* points are the metal, water, wood, fire, and earth points respectively.

This twofold knowledge of how to predict the number of the *Jing* (well), *Ying* (spring), and *Shu* (stream) points on a meridian, as well as how to assign elemental energies to them, is a useful skill that allows us to further understand the elemental function of a point.

Also, understanding the elemental energy of the points fulfills several other important functions. First, it provides an appreciation of the basic energetic configuration of that point. For instance, HT 9 (*Shaochong*) is the wood point on a fire meridian. As such, it can be used to add or delete wood energy from the fire meridian. The nature of the wood element should come to mind here, that is, the point has a woody, regenerative, spring-like quality to it. Secondly, the elemental energy of a point is not only related to the energy incarnated in that point but also to the meridian the point is on.

To continue with the example of HT 9 (*Shaochong*), the wood point on a fire meridian, the relationship between wood and fire is one of nourishment, promotion, and growth. It is what we would call the tonification or mother point of the meridian. Thus, HT 9 (*Shaochong*) can be used to tonify the Heart meridian–organ. Tonification and dispersion points are primary treatment sites on any meridian for building or reducing the energy in the organ–meridian complex. It is through the coupling of an elemental point with proper needle technique that the tonification or dispersion is accomplished.

An example of a dispersion point on the Heart meridian would be HT 7 (*Shenmen*), the *Shu* (stream) point and the earth point. First, earth points assist in balancing; they can add or take away earth energy from the element in question and we can use the point in this way. Second, the relationship between earth and fire is one of the son (earth) who receives or takes energy from the mother (fire). This is called the dispersion or sedation point. When this point is needled with a dispersion technique it can balance the Heart and take excess earth energy from the Heart meridian–organ such as Dampness or Phlegm.

There is another interesting elemental relationship when the point in question has the same elemental energy as the meridian it is located on. An example of this is HT 8 (*Shaofu*), the fire point on a fire meridian. The term for this type of point is the Horary point. Horary points always manifest the same elemental energy as the meridian they are on. In this case HT 8 (*Shaofu*) is a very "fiery" point. It can be used to add or take away fire from the meridian. Table 8.4 records the Tonification, Dispersion, and Horary points of the Twelve Main Meridians, and Table 8.5 lists the points that correspond to each element.

Table 8.4. The Tonification, Dispersion, and Horary
Points of the Twelve Main Meridians

Meridian	Tonification	Dispersion	Horary
Lung	LU 9	LU 5	LU 8
Large Intestine	LI 11	LI 2	LI 1
Stomach	ST 41	ST 45	ST 36
Spleen	SP 2	SP 5	SP 3

(continued)

Meridian	Tonification	Dispersion	Horary
Heart	HT 9	HT 7	HT 8
Small Intestine	SI 3	SI 8	SI 5
Bladder	BL 67	BL 65	BL 66
Kidney	KI 7	KI 1	KI 10
Pericardium	PC 9	PC 7	PC 8
Triple Burner	TB 3	TB 10	TB 6
Gall Bladder	GB 43	GB 38	GB 41
Liver	LR 8	LR 2	LR 1

Table 8.5. The Elemental Energy of the Points

Meridian	Wood	Fire	Earth	Metal	Water
Lung	11	10	9	8	5
Large Intestine	3	5	11	1	2
Stomach	43	41	36	45	44
Spleen	1	2	3	5	9
Heart	9	8	7	4	3
Small Intestine	3	5	8	1	2
Bladder	65	60	40	67	66
Kidney	1	2	3	7	10
Pericardium	9	8	7	5	3
Triple Burner	3	6	10	1	2
Gall Bladder	41	38	34	44	43
Liver	1	2	3	4	8

Finally *Shu* points can be used seasonally in a very literal sense of the Five Element season from spring to winter. For instance, in the spring, allergy symptoms that can cause asthma are common as the season is typically windy and allergens travel on the wind. Thus a *Jing* (well) point such as LU 11(*Shaoshang*) might be useful to regulate asthmatic cough.

The *Shu* points can also be used for their figurative association with a season, meaning the early (spring) to deep (winter) of a disorder. For instance, just as a *Jing* (well) point is like a bubbling of water in a well, or a *Ying* spring point is like a spring, each can be used for a certain stage of a disease from an early stage like the *Jing* (well), to a deep organ stage like the *He* (sea). Additionally, there are six Lower *He* (sea) points, which are related to the *Fu* organs. When a *Fu* organ is affected, Lower *He* (sea) points may be indicated for use.

Table 8.6, The Use of the Command Points for the Seasonal Treatment of Disease, specifically illustrates a classical method of using the Five *Shu* points seasonally in both a literal and figurative manner.

Table 8.6. The Use of the Command Points for the Seasonal Treatment of Disease

Shu Point	*Jing* (Well)	*Ying* (Spring)	*Shu* (Stream)	*Jing* (River)	*He* (Sea)
Seasonal usage	The season of spring, as well as the *spring* of the disease	Summer or the *summer* of the disease	Late summer or the *late summer* of the disease	Fall or the *fall* of the disease	Winter or the *winter* of the disease
Clinical manifestations	Mental disorders, chest disorders, coma, unconsciousness, stifling sensation in chest, acute problems, apparent fullness, first aid, *Yin* organ problems	Fevers, febrile diseases	Painful joints caused by pathogenic heat and Damp, *Yin* organ problems	Asthma, throat, cough disorders, alternating chills and fever, muscle and bone problems	Disorders of the *Fu* organs, bleeding Stomach, diarrhea (tends not to affect the meridian at this level)

2. Yuan (Source) points

Each of the twelve main meridians has a *Yuan* (Source) point located bilaterally on the extremities. As the name implies, they are points where Source energy, the original *Qi* of inherited essence, is stored, pooled, and may be accessed. They are responsible for the regulation of the Source *Qi* and this property makes then closely connected to the

Triple Burner system. They are very effective points for both diagnosis and treatment because of this property.

The *Yuan* (Source) points stimulate the vital energy of the twelve main meridians, regulate the functional activities of the internal organs, reinforce the antipathogenic factor which is the True *Qi* of the body, and eliminate pathogenic causes of disease. They are useful points for treating the root of a problem, particularly disorders of the internal organs. They are generally used for chronic problems. As such, I term them foundational points that reinforce the foundational energy of the body.

The Source point of a meridian has a strong relationship to the *Luo* point of its coupled meridian. Because of this relationship, the coupled meridian's *Luo* point can tap into some of this consigned essence. How to use *Luo* points in clinical strategies is discussed in Chapter 15.

Just as the *Jing* (well) points and the *Ying* (spring) points are always the first- and second-most distal points on a meridian respectively, the Source point is invariably the third-most distal point on a *Yin* meridian. LU 9 (*Taiyuan*), HT 7 (*Shenmen*), and SP 3 (*Taibai*) are examples of this rule. On a *Yin* meridian the *Shu* (stream) point and the *Yuan* (Source) point are the same point, thus making these points more potent.

On a *Yang* meridian, the fourth-most distal point, with the exception of the Gall Bladder meridian, is always the *Yuan* (Source) point. Thus, LI 4 (*Hegu*), SI 4 (*Wangu*), and BL 64 (*Jinggu*) are Source points.

3. *Luo* (connecting) points

A *Luo* point is a special vessel of communication between vessels. Each of the twelve main meridians possesses a *Luo* point. In addition, the Conception and the Governing Vessel channels each have a *Luo* point. The Spleen has two *Luo* points, its regular *Luo* point SP 4 (*Gongsun*), and another SP 21 (*Dabao*), known as the Grand *Luo*, which goes to the hypochondriac region and connects all the *Luo* points as well as the blood vessels. Some sources claim that ST 18 (*Rugen*) is a second *Luo* point on the Stomach meridian that connects the Stomach to the Heart.

Luo points can be used in two ways, either as transverse or longitudinal vessels. In treatment, the way to differentiate a longitudinal *Luo* from a transverse *Luo* is by the angle of insertion of the needle.

Therefore, the importance of correct needle technique cannot be overestimated for achieving the desired therapeutic result.

A transverse *Luo* sends a stimulus directly to the *Yuan* (Source) point of its coupled organ. For instance, when we stimulate LI 6 (*Pianli*), the *Luo* point of the Large Intestine meridian, it sends energy to its coupled Source point, LU 9 (*Taiyuan*). This technique links the internal–external meridians together, that is, it connects the coupled organ–meridian *Yin/Yang* complexes in the Five Element system. The effect of such a treatment plan is to create a homeostatic connection between the two coupled meridians so that, for example, Large Intestine energy can be tapped and brought to the Lung meridian, thus harmonizing that pair.

A longitudinal *Luo* links with its corresponding organ, and stimulates that organ. In the same way, when it is needled longitudinally, LI 6 (*Pianli*) sends a stimulus to the Large Intestine organ–meridian itself. In this case, the Large Intestine meridian–organ is stimulated directly instead of Large Intestine energy being borrowed to stimulate Lung function as in the previous illustration. A transverse *Luo* can be needled in several directions. This strategy is discussed in the needle technique chapter on *Luos*, Chapter 15.

There are other *Luos* that do not connect *Yin/Yang* couples together, such as the *Bao Luo*, a special communication vessel between the Kidney and the uterus; the *Luo* of the Conception Vessel channel, which connects to the abdomen and dominates the collaterals of the *Yin* channels; the *Luo* of the Governing Vessel channel, which goes to the head and dominates the collaterals of the *Yang* channels; and the Grand *Luo* of the Spleen, which goes to the hypochondriac region and connects all of the *Luo* points as well as the blood vessels.

In addition, there are four group *Luos*: SP 6 (*Sanyinjiao*), the group *Luo* of the Three Leg *Yin*; GB 39 (*Xuanzhong*), group *Luo* of the Three Leg *Yang*; PC 5 (*Jianshi*), group *Luo* of the Three Arm *Yin*; and TE 8 (*Sanyangluo*), group *Luo* of the Three Arm *Yang*. These group *Luos*, because of their multiple intersections, are strong points for activating the energy of the meridians they control. Chapter 15 fully explains and includes various opinions on the use of *Luo* points both theoretically and practically coordinated with the correct needle technique.

4. Entry and exit points

Another way in which energy flows between meridians is through their entry and exit points. Table 8.1 previously referenced on the Points of the Fourteen Channels illustrates the entry and exit points.

5. *Xi* (cleft) points

As the name implies, *Xi* (cleft) points are points where the *Qi* of the channel is deeply converged in a cleft. There are sixteen *Xi* (cleft) points: one from each of the twelve main meridians and four from certain Curious Vessels. A perusal of the insertion depths for acupuncture points along a meridian shows that typically they are slightly deeper for a *Xi* (cleft) point than for adjacent points along the same meridian. Figure 8.1, Location of *Xi* (Cleft) Points, illustrates the location of *Xi* (cleft) points.

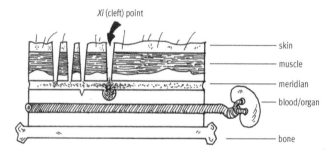

Figure 8.1: Location of Xi *(Cleft) Points*

Xi (cleft) points are located on the extremities, that is, below the knees or above the elbow with the exception of ST 34 (*Liangqiu*). ST 34 (*Liangqiu*) is the only *Xi* (cleft) point located above the knees. *Xi* (cleft) points are considered to be meridian reflex points, meaning that they show the health or dysfunction of a meridian. When palpated, or observed for abnormal colorations, they can be used as diagnostic points of the meridians. *Xi* (cleft) points are utilized for acute disorders that manifest as pain, accumulation, stagnation, and inflammation in an area. For instance, ST 34 (*Liangqiu*) is beneficial for stomachache and SP 8 (*Diji*) for menstrual cramps. *Xi* (cleft) points can be used for any inflammation. This usage is a critical strategy for pain and blockage. There are four *Xi* (cleft) points, utilized in the same manner, that correspond to four of the Eight Extra meridians. They are found in Table 8.3, previously referenced. Chapter 18 discusses needling techniques for *Xi* (cleft) points.

6. Front *Mu* points

Front *Mu* points, also known as Alarm points or Front Collecting points, are of the utmost clinical significance in the point classification system. There are twelve Front *Mu* points all located on the chest and abdomen, each related to one of the twelve main meridians.

Because the Front *Mu* points are close to their respective organs, it is not surprising that the *Qi*, which is the *Yin* and *Yang* of the *Zang-fu* organs bound together, is infused in these points. They are particularly reactive to pathological changes in the body and when the organs are affected, these points become tender.

Front *Mu* points, very important in diagnosis and treatment, are particularly valuable in the treatment of chronic disorders. They reveal the *Yin/Yang* disharmony of each organ and, as the classics tell us, when the six *Fu* are diseased, the *Yang* diseases devolve to their *Yin* aspect, meaning we can diagnose them on the front of the body. See Table 8.7 for the Front *Mu* points and their needling methods and angles and depths of insertion.

Table 8.7. The Front *Mu* Points and Needle Techniques

	Organ	Points	Needle Technique
1.	LU	LU 1	0.5–0.8 obliquely laterally
2.	PC	CV 17	0.3–0.5 subcutaneously upward
3.	HT	CV15	0.4–0.6 p or obliquely upward
4.	ST	CV 12	0.5–1.2 p
5.	LI	ST 25	0.7–1.2 p
6.	TB	CV 5	0.5–1.0 p
7.	SI	CV 4	0.8–1.2 p
8.	BL	CV 3	0.5–1.0 p
9.	GB	GB 24	0.3–0.5 o

(continued)

	Organ	Points	Needle Technique
10.	LR	LR 14	0.3–0.8 o
11.	SP	LR 13	0.5–0.8 p
12.	KI	GB 25	0.3–0.5 p

p = perpendicularly
o = obliquely

7. Back *Shu* points

Back *Shu* points, also called Associated points or Back Transforming points, are located on the dorsal or back surface of the body close to their respective organs and parallel to the vertebral column. The *Qi* and *Blood* of the organs are infused in the Back *Shu* points, thus they are particularly helpful in distinguishing *Qi* and *Blood* pathology. The Front *Mu* points, in contrast, are better for discriminating *Yin* and *Yang* disharmonies. Back *Shu* points are useful for chronic illness.

There are twelve pairs of Back *Shu* points, one pair for each of the twelve *Zang-fu* organs, and also for a number of other organs and structures, for instance the diaphragm and the lumbar vertebrae. See Table 8.8, The Back *Shu* Points and Needle Techniques, for the needling technique and angles and depths of insertions of the Back *Shu* points.

Table 8.8. The Back *Shu* Points and Needle Techniques

	Organs	Points	Needle Technique	Vertebral Level
1.	LU	BL 13	0.5–0.7 o m	T3
2.	PC	BL 14	0.5–0.7 o m	T4
3.	HT	BL 15	0.5–0.7 o m	T5
4.	LR	BL 18	0.5–0.7 o m	T9
5.	GB	BL 19	0.5–0.8 o m	T10
6.	SP	BL 20	0.5–0.7 o m	T11
7.	ST	BL 21	0.5–0.8 o m	T12
8.	TB	BL 22	0.5–1 p	L1
9.	KI	BL 23	1–1.2 p	L2
10.	LI	BL 25	0.8–1.2 p	L5

11.	ST	BL 27	0.8–1.2 p	S1
12.	BL	BL 28	0.8–1.2 p	S3

p = perpendicularly
o = obliquely
m = medially

Table 8.9 lists the Front *Mu* and Back *Shu* points of the twelve main meridians, the organs, and structures for discriminating *Yin/Yang* and *Qi* and *Blood* disharmonies respectively.

Table 8.9. The Front *Mu* and Back *Shu* Points

Meridian/Organ/Structure	Front *Mu*	Back *Shu*
Lung	LU 1	BL 13
Large Intestine	ST 25	BL 25
Stomach	CV 12	BL 21
Spleen	LR 13	BL 20
Heart	CV 15	BL 15
Small Intestine	CV 4	BL 27
Bladder	CV 3	BL 28
Kidney	GB 25	BL 23
Pericardium	CV 17	BL 14
Triple Burner	CV 5	BL 22
Gall Bladder	GB 24	BL 19
Liver	LR 14	BL 18
Governing Vessel	X	BL 16
Conception Vessel	X	X
Bones	X	BL 11
Upper Lung	X	BL 12
Diaphragm	X	BL 17
Lumbar vertebrae	X	BL 24
Lower lumbar area	X	BL 26
Sacrum	X	BL 29
Bladder sphincter	X	BL 30

8. The Eight Influential points

The Eight Influential points are a noteworthy group of points that exert special influence on their associated entities. Sometimes they are called the Eight Influential points of the Eight Tissues. Additionally, these points have other important energetics that enhance their status. The Eight Influential points and what they dominate are found in Table 8.10.

Table 8.10. The Eight Influential Points

Point	Area of Influence	Point	Area of Influence
LR 13	*Zang* organs	LU 9	Vessels
CV 12	*Fu* organs	GB 39	*Marrow*
BL 17	*Blood*	CV 17	*Qi*
GB 34	Tendons	BL 11	Bone

9. Confluent points

The Eight Confluent points, also known as Master points, refer to the points of each of the Eight Curious Vessels that activate the physiology pertaining to those vessels. In addition, each Curious Vessel also has a Coupled point, that is, a point that when activated, works well with its corresponding meridian. Although certain Curious Vessels operate well in pairs, they can also be used separately to treat disorders of the corresponding meridian. Chapter 16 discusses the use of the Eight Curious Vessels. The Confluent points are strong points for treatment because of their connection with the Eight Curious Vessels in addition to the fact that these points also control other significant energetics. Table 8.11, The Master and Coupled Points of the Eight Curious Vessels, lists the Eight Curious Vessels along with their Master and Coupled points.

Table 8.11. The Master and Coupled Points of the Eight Curious Vessels

Meridian	Master Point	Coupled Point
Governing Vessel (GV)	SI 3	BL 62
Conception Vessel (CV)	LU 7	KI 6

Chong (TV)	SP 4	PC 6
Dai (DV)	GB 41	TB 5
Yinqiao (YINHV)	KI 6	LU 7
Yangqiao (YANGHV)	BL 62	SI 3
Yinwei (YINLV)	PC 6	SP 4
Yangwei (YANGLV)	TB 5	GB 41

10. Coalescent points

Coalescent points are defined as points of intersection between the Eight Curious Vessels and the twelve main meridians. As has been obvious throughout this discussion, the greater the range of energetics of a point, the greater its clinical utility. Examples of Coalescent points include BL 1 (Qingming), the intersection of the Bladder and Yangqiao meridians; GB 20 (Fengchi), the intersection of the Gall Bladder, Yangwei, and Yangqiao meridians; and ST 8 (Touwei), intersection of the Stomach and Yangwei meridians. Other Coalescent points can be found in most standard texts.

11. Crossing points

Crossing points, also referred to as Union points or points of Reunion, represent points of intersection between two or more main channels. Most of these ninety points are located on the head, face, and trunk. They are very efficient points to use because of their multiple intersections of the two or more meridians that cross. Examples of important Crossing points include CV 3 (Zhongji), meeting of the Three Leg Yin on the abdomen, and ST 13 (Qihu), meeting of the Stomach, Large Intestine, and Triple Burner meridians. Other Crossing points can be found in most standard point location books.

12. The Four Command points

The Four Command points influence certain areas of the body such as the head and neck, face and mouth, and back and abdomen.

The four Command points are ST 36 (*Zusanli*) for the abdomen, BL 40 (*Weizhong*) for the back, LU 7 *(Lieque)* for the head and neck, and LI 4 (*Hegu*) for the mouth and face.

13. Tendinomuscular meridian points

The tendinomuscular meridian points aid in muscular, skin, and pain problems. They are GB 22 (*Yuanye*) for the arm *Yin*, CV 3 (*Zhongji*) and CV 4 (*Guanyuan*) for the leg *Yin*, GB 13 (*Benshen*) and ST 8 (*Touwei*) for the arm *Yang*, and ST 2 (*Sibai*) and SI 18 (*Quanliao*) for the leg *Yang*.

14. Window to the Sky points

This special group of points affects disorders of *Qi* and *Blood* flow to the head. They include the following:

- ST 9 (*Renying*): best point to control *Qi* flow to the head

- LI 18 (*Futu*): sends a vessel to the tongue, for speech problems

- TE 16 (*Tianyu*): for dizziness, facial swelling, blurry vision, sudden deafness

- BL 10 (*Tianshu*): relaxes the sympathetic nervous system, increases vasodilation

- LU 3 (*Sanjian*): increases oxygenation to the brain and the body

The Extra points

The Extra points, also known as the non-meridian points, are points that have definite locations and known energetics but that are not located along the course of a main meridian. They number in the hundreds and are specified by name or number, for example, *Taiyang* or M-HN-9 (Bensky and O'Connor 1981). Functionally, they are useful points to supplement the points of the fourteen channels. They have been discovered by clinical experience and hence may also be called Clinically Effective points.

The *Ah Shi* points

The *Ah Shi* points are tender points. When palpated the person says "Oh, yes!" (*Ah Shi*). They are points that either fire spontaneously, or are discovered by palpation or other mechanical means such as an electropoint detector. Their number is virtually unlimited because any place on the body can be a tender point. They do not have definite locations or names.

Summary

In addition to how points are classified, each point is significantly named and the point's use can be related to its name. A perusal of their translations shows that points are named in various ways. Some points' names carry an analogy to the earth, such as mountains and valleys. BL 60 (*Kunlun*), Kunlun Mountains, and LI 4 (*Hegu*), Meeting of the Valleys, are examples of this. Other points like LU 10 (*Yuji*), Fish Border, are analogous to animals. Architectural structures and astronomical and meteorological phenomena are represented in points such as CV 22 (*Tiantu*), Heaven Chimney, GV 23 (*Shangxing*), Upper Star, and GB 20 (*Fengchi*), Wind Pool. CV 12 (*Zhongwan*), Middle Stomach, ST 1 (*Chengqi*), Receives Tears, and CV 9 (*Shuifen*), Separates the Clear from the Turbid indicate anatomical terms, therapeutic properties, and physiological/pathological changes. *Yin/Yang* properties and theories of *Zang-fu* and meridians are expressed in points such as GB 34 (*Yanglingquan*), Source of the *Yang* Mountain, and SP 6 (*Sanyinjiao*), Crossroad of Three *Yin*.

Certainly there is no shortage of acupuncture books that provide various versions of the translated names of the points. Although all translations are subjective, they range from literal rigidity to loosely figurative interpretations. Some translations achieve a functional and insightful balance between the two extremes. The practitioner is encouraged to read books and consult other sources that can provide point names that will assist in understanding point function.

Case 2 provides a clinical example of one highly underutilized, yet effective type of acupuncture point.

CASE 2: NUMBNESS TREATED THROUGH THE *JING* (WELL) POINTS

The patient's major complaint was one-sided numbness in the distal phalanxes of his thumb and index finger. This condition was accompanied by an electrical sensation that would occur when he lifted his arms over his head. The patient is a bronze worker who sits in a hunched position over his work that requires extremely fine and controlled hand movements. Overwork, stretching, and heavy work, such as yard work, aggravated his hand when his shoulders and arms were used excessively. He had received no Western medical diagnosis, although his condition resembled neurovascular compression of the brachial plexus.

The tongue was pale purple, flabby, scalloped, and slightly deviated to the left. The coat was wet, thick, yellow, and greasy. There were red dots on the tip, as well as cracks in the Lung area. The pulse was in the middle to superficial position, wiry, excessive, and fast. His Chinese diagnosis was *Qi* and *Blood* deficiency in the Lung and Large Intestine channels. The etiology was due to neurovascular compression or deficiency of the channels due to postural stress as well as an underlying Heart *Qi* deficiency.

Points were needled along the course of the affected channels of the Lung and Large Intestine meridians, specifically LU 9 (*Taiyuan*), the influential point that dominates the vessels, and their *Jing* (well) points, LU 11 (*Shaoshang*) and LI 1 (*Shangyang*) to activate the *Qi* and *Blood*. The *Shixuan* points of the thumb and index finger were also needled. In addition, a distal point, ST 12 (*Quepen*), was also treated to alleviate the neurovascular compression that was occurring because of occupationally induced poor posture.

After the first treatment, the numbness in the hand was immediately better. Feeling was restored to the thumb. Because of the patient's schedule, the next treatment was administered in two weeks. Following the second treatment, feeling was restored to both fingers.

Conscious postural improvement, the needle schema, and the application of *Zheng Gu Shui*, the deepest penetrating Chinese liniment, along the course of the involved meridians to activate the flow of *Qi* and *Blood* completely resolved the numbness in five treatments. The patient was extremely satisfied with the results and was able to renew his work with no further or future impairment.

We should note that occupation and constitution might interfere with long-lasting results. The patient needs to be more conscious about his postural tension, which contributes to his major complaint. However, there are other constitutional weaknesses that were revealed during the interview that if strengthened, could enhance the effects of treatment. Such weaknesses include a history of heart disease and hypertension in the family. However, the patient preferred to end the course of treatment because of monetary considerations and the fact that he was satisfied with the treatment results for which he sought assistance.

Chapter 9

The Rules of Point Selection and General Treatment Strategies

Learning Objectives

In this chapter the readers will gain information by which to organize their treatments. The order of needle insertion is never arbitrary but grounded in principles of Chinese medical theory, although they are seldom articulated. Their implementation makes a difference in the execution and efficacy of the treatment.

In Chapter 8, I discussed how to select points based on the Chinese point classification system. In particular, that chapter outlined the potency of each particular category of points. In connection with the Command points, through the analogy of different bodies of water, I discussed the amount and type of *Qi* contained in each of these points. In addition, I discussed how to use these points seasonally, both in a literal and figurative sense. A discussion of how to select points for treatment is beneficial to beginning students of Chinese medicine, who usually lack the breadth and depth of clinical experience to support their choice of points, yet even advanced clinicians may not be aware of the unarticulated "rules" of point selection. The outline that follows presents the parameters and the options for selecting points for treatment and their order of insertion.

As students of Chinese medicine are well aware, it is customary in acupuncture colleges to receive copious clinical indications compiled by practitioners from varied sources such as their teachers and textbooks. However, without a sense of how points are classified and organized, students depend on memorizing or consulting notes instead of utilizing a thinking process that is more in accord with the artistry of the diagnostic process and the patient's presentation. Neither of these can be found in any text. There are as many treatment options as there are patients and for that reason thinking and attentiveness must guide the practitioner to the correct treatment plan. Table 9.1 on the Rules of Point Selection highlights a dozen different approaches that summarize the ways practitioners can think about how to select points for treatment. Concomitantly, there are several different ways to execute needling strategy that practitioners should keep in mind. Needle placement is never arbitrary; it is part of a treatment plan that should be executed in a logical and methodical order based on the aim of treatment as expressed in the treatment plan.

Table 9.1. The Rules of Point Selection

How to Select Points for Clinical Use
Command points Seasonal disturbances (see Table 8.6) Classical Antique point usage (see Table 8.3)
Essential substance pathology (*Qi*, *Blood*, *Jin-ye*, *Jing*, *Shen*, and *Marrow* deficiencies, stagnation, imbalances)
Unique energetics of each point
Name of the point
Pathway of the meridian
Chinese physiology and pathology (for instance, to treat Stomach ulcer, the Lung point in the ear is effective because the Lung controls mucous membranes and ulcers affect the mucous membranes)
Local and distal points
Five Seas (Nourishment, *Blood*, *Qi*, *Marrow*, and Internal Pollution)
Functional phases of points (active, passive, latent)
Organ–Meridian symptomatology
Organ interrelationships (therapeutic properties of the coupled channels in various diagnostic paradigms)
Understanding of Western science (anatomy, physiology, pathology)

THE RULES OF POINT SELECTION

1. Command points can be used for "seasonal" disturbances as well as for their classical Antique point usage. An example of using a point seasonally would be to use LU 11 (*Shaoshang*). This point, the wood point on a metal meridian, can be needled for the "spring" of a condition, that is, one that has come on quickly or actually in the season of spring such as allergies. In this case, wood energy is excessive and is failing to control the *Blood*, leading to symptoms of *Blood* extravasation occurring in the metal meridian, on which it is counteracting. *Blood* problems in the physiological domains that metal governs such as the nose, throat, and chest may cause pathological conditions such as epistaxis and hemoptysis.

2. Points can be selected that treat the pathologies of the essential substances of *Qi*, *Blood*, *Jin-ye*, *Jing*, *Shen*, *Marrow* with their deficiencies, stagnations, rebelliousness, or sinkingness. For example, CV 6 (*Qihai*) can be used to tonify Kidney *Qi* deficiency.

3. Points have peculiar, special energetics that distinguish them from other points; for example, GV 20 (*Baihui*) raises sinking Spleen *Qi*.

4. The names of the points suggest ways in which to use them. For example, SP 6 (*Sanyinjiao*) is the meeting of the Three Leg *Yin* meridians and those three meridians can be effectively treated through this point.

5. The pathway of the meridian, which has both internal and external manifestations, can be used as the basis for point consideration. For example, CV 12 (*Zhongwan*) is a possible point for treatment of vertical headache because the internal Liver meridian ends at CV 12 (*Zhongwan*) and Liver headaches typically manifest at the top of the head.

6. An understanding of Chinese physiology and pathology provides unique insights into the functioning of the human body and how to treat it with certain points. For example, to treat a Stomach ulcer, the Lung point in the ear is extremely

effective because according to *Zang-fu* theory, the Lung controls the mucous membranes and the Stomach ulcer is a problem in the wearing down of the inner mucosa of the Stomach.

7. For excess conditions, a combination of local and distal points is an effective treatment strategy. For example, select Command points that are major distal points for an area of dysfunction. Select local points such as *Mu* or *Shu* points that are close to an organ and the sphere of energy that it controls. In the case of migraine, for instance, GB 41 (*Zulinqi*), a distal point, with GB 20 (*Fengchi*), a local point, is a good combination.

8. Activate the Five Seas, which pertain to energetic zones of the body. The Five Seas and the level of the body they are involved with are important points:

    •   The Sea of Nourishment assists in food absorption. It can be activated when the person has overeaten or is hungry or undernourished. Its points are ST 30 (*Qichong*) and ST 36 (*Zusanli*).

    •   The Sea of Blood can tonify deficient *Blood* or move *Blood* stagnation. The Sea of Blood points are ST 37 (*Shangjuxu*), BL 11 (*Dazhu*), SP 10 (*Xuehai*), BL 17 (*Geshu*), and ST 39 (*Xiajuxu*).

    •   Immediately usable points, reservoirs of energy that can be tapped, activate the Sea of Energy, also referred to as the Sea of *Qi*. They are CV 6 (*Qihai*), ST 9 (*Renying*), CV 17 (*Tanzhong*), BL 10 (*Tianzhu*), and GV 14 (*Dazhui*).

    •   The Sea of Marrow assists in strengthening the brain and the mind. Its points include GB 39 (*Xuanzhong*), GV 15 (*Yamen*), GV 16 (*Fengfu*), and GV 20 (*Baihui*).

    •   The Sea of Internal Pollution refers to organs that help the body rid itself of waste. They are the Lung, Kidney, Bladder, and Large Intestine organs. Use their respective points.

9. Points possess various functional phases that are manifestations of their health. Active points are those that are active or that

fire spontaneously because of their pathology. They represent a problem in the physiology of a particular point. For example, a pre-appendicitis condition may be detected by a throbbing sensation at *Lanwei*, the appendix reflex point, or pain in the ST 25 (*Tianshu*) area, close by the appendix. Likewise, sinus congestion may be signified by pressure in the BL 2 (*Zanzhu*), ST 1 (*Chengqi*), and ST 2 (*Sibai*) areas.

10. Passive points are those points that only react when they are mechanically stimulated or aroused through pressure. For example, a patient with Spleen *Qi* deficiency and Damp generally has exquisite tenderness when palpated at SP 4 (*Gongsun*) whether the manifestations of Spleen *Qi* deficiency with Damp are overt or preclinical.

11. Latent points are those points that are neither active nor passive, that is, they are not spontaneously painful or painful when palpated. They indicate that the function of each point is healthy and not a problem. The more latent points there are, the healthier the person is. These points can be selected to enhance bodily function.

12. Specific organ–meridian symptomatology is clearly associated with each organ–meridian complex that suggests point use. For instance, the Large Intestine organ–meridian complex clearly deals with intestinal problems. Likewise, because the channel traverses the shoulder area, LI 15 (*Jianyu*) can be used for shoulder problems and LI 4 (*Hegu*) is indicated for tooth problems because its meridian traverses the mouth area.

13. The therapeutic properties of a point may be modified by the organ–meridian complex it is coupled with. For example:

   • The Lung meridian may be treated alone.

   • The Lung meridian may be treated in combination with the Large Intestine because of its Five Element relationship.

   • The Lung meridian may be combined with the Spleen meridian by virtue of its Six Division association.

- The Lung meridian may be used with the Kidney meridian because of extraordinary meridian and *Zang-fu* energetics, for instance the Lung is the mother of Kidney.

14. An understanding of Western anatomy, physiology, pathology, and other clinical sciences can shed light on point selection. For example, ST 36 (*Zusanli*) can be chosen to adjust indigestion from excess or deficient hydrochloric acid secretion.

SELECTION OF TREATMENT STRATEGIES

The aforementioned list of possibilities does not imply that only one paradigm can be chosen when a treatment plan of points is being generated. Rather, it simply gives some guidelines to assist the practitioner in choosing points. The process of initiating treatment is a highly logical procedure within the Chinese healthcare delivery system. Point selection follows the treatment plan, which follows diagnosis. But diagnosis is a highly sophisticated art involving the synthesis of all of the data gained by asking questions, palpating the pulse and the body, auscultation, olfaction, inspection, and numerous other parameters. This integration, while logical, is both artful and intuitive in the sense that intuition is knowledge based upon the integration of perceptions.

Beginning students of Oriental medicine can be overwhelmed by all the methods that can be used to establish the basis for a diagnosis, never mind the complexity of weaving that information into a whole that addresses the person's problem. Students assiduously strive to cover everything that must be mastered in order to know as much as possible about the person, and this is learned well in schools. What takes longer, and what is generally only grasped in clinical practice, is where to begin with the treatment of the person, how to capture the essence of the person, the root of the problem, and the way in which to initiate the treatment process. This ability may be a function of experience and alacrity on the part of the observant practitioner who attunes the individual presence of the patient to her or his own individual skill as a physician. However, a few general treatment principles can be advanced for the practitioners of Oriental medicine and these can assist the practitioner and the patient in their discovery of balance.

1. The first and golden rule of medical ethics and treatment is always to do no harm. This maxim demands much skill, honesty, precision, and humbleness on the part of practitioners to treat what they are comfortable in treating. There must also be an awareness of the seriousness of illness, their own scope of knowledge and practice, and an understanding of the intricacies of organ interrelationships, needle technique, point location, herbal, dietary, and other lifestyle considerations. There must be integrity of spirit and a willingness to learn and develop skills to meet ever changing medical problems and the complexity and uniqueness of each individual patient. There must be total attentiveness and mindfulness during every step of the intake and the delivery system and knowledge of when to refer to other healthcare providers if the case exceeds the practitioner's ability to treat.

2. No harmful treatment should ever be administered. If the practitioner treats to the best of their ability with this guideline "to do no harm" in mind, they will encompass the spirit of a physician. Many times "doing no harm" for the average practitioner means to not do too much in a treatment, that is, over-treating with too many needles or adjunct therapies. Yet doing no harm implies doing what the practitioner should be able to accomplish through their education, that is, the practitioner needs technical competency. The other part of this maxim to do no harm, is its correlate—to do the best we can—which is what the patient expects of medical providers.

3. With these guidelines as the automatic operating assumptions on the part of the patient and the practitioner, practitioners then need to formulate an overall strategy with which to accomplish their objectives. Point selection and needling strategies must be adopted if acupuncture is part of the therapeutic modality. Practitioners have numerous historical positions from which to adopt a treatment strategy. Table 9.2 summarizes the needle strategies that can be considered after point selection has occurred.

Table 9.2. Needling Strategies

Treat both the major complaint and the accompanying symptoms within the context of the whole person: • Know when to treat the acute condition, when to treat the chronic, when the acute is a manifestation of the chronic, that is: when to treat the root, or treat the branch, or treat the root and the branch • While reinforcing the root, concentrate on it yet don't be too redundant • Know when to disperse a pathogenic factor, when to reduce • Know when to strengthen the body, when to reinforce • Differentiate the problem with the diagnostic framework of choice
Be efficient with point selection
Choose clinically effective points
Generally, insert needles from top to bottom to bring the energy down. In emergency conditions, however, sometimes the energy needs to be raised, and then the needles are inserted from bottom to top
Insert needles from front to back, from right to left, from the midline to the lateral aspect. This brings the *Yin* into the *Yang*. Remove needles in the order that they were inserted
Insert needles singularly for their known abilities
Insert needles in a chain of points
Encircle a point with needles
Needle the points on the upper extremities first, then on the lower, and from exterior to interior to bring the *Yang* to the interior (*Yin*). This action will tonify

NEEDLING STRATEGIES

Three major orientations cover all the diseases that will be clinically encountered. They are treating the root, treating the branch (manifestation), and treating both the root and the branch:

1. Treating the root is perhaps the purest of all treatment strategies. It embodies the Chinese emphasis on ameliorating the underlying problem in order to restore the patient to balance. This approach can be used especially if the clinical signs and symptoms are not severe or immediately life threatening. There are numerous treatment styles within this approach and all aim

at correcting the root imbalance. These styles include balancing the pulses, eliminating navel tension, or reducing the number of passive and active points in the body. Although the scope of this book is not to outline how the root is perceived or corrected in the individual, it is the thesis of this book that failure to treat the root or foundational energy in many cases represents a symptomatic approach to medicine and may provide only minimal relief. Our goal is foremost to treat the foundational energies of the patient from which the symptoms arise.

2. Treating the branch, that is, the manifestations, has its place in the scheme of treatment. This is a beneficial and indeed appropriate treatment strategy when the problem is acute and/ or life threatening in nature. The patient's problem demands that it be dealt with immediately. This approach necessitates a spirit of compassion and an ability to perceive the causes of signs and symptoms. It is Chinese emergency medicine at its best.

3. Treat the root and treat the branch manifestation is an effective treatment plan that is used most often by most practitioners. This approach simultaneously acknowledges both the presenting complaint of the person as well as the root cause of the disorder. It is used for chronic conditions and constitutes an efficient treatment strategy as long as the practitioner has the ability to see how the manifestations of the symptoms are connected to the root of the problem of the foundational energy.

Regardless of which approach is selected, all treatment styles require that both the major complaint and the accompanying symptoms be addressed within the context of the whole person. The practitioner must learn to discern when to treat the acute condition, when to treat chronic conditions, and when the acute is a manifestation of the underlying, chronic problem. As in good herbal medicine, points are chosen for how they work together to treat the pattern of the illness. Neither points nor herbs should be used to treat each sign and symptom without considering the whole pattern.

Other treatment approaches are important to bear in mind as well. Skilled practitioners who do no harm and also do the best they can must have the wisdom to know when to disperse a pathogenic factor and when to strengthen the body, that is, when to reinforce, when to reduce, and when not to be redundant. They must be able to discern whether the problem is one of the *Zang-fu*, the essential substances, and so on. Once a proper differentiation is made based on the theoretical framework that the practitioner adopts, a treatment plan must be formulated that matches the chosen diagnostic framework and the related, selected points. Needle technique must match the treatment plan.

For beginning students of acupuncture, this step oftentimes feels overwhelming. It can be difficult to know what is going on with the patient when so much information needs to be assimilated. Two major pitfalls that students can succumb to are what can be called the shotgun approach on the one hand, and tunnel vision on the other.

With the shotgun approach, instead of a precise, discerning diagnosis, there is a tendency to think that everything is involved. Because it is difficult for beginning practitioners to see the bigger picture of patterns and interrelationships their treatment strategies tend to be imprecise and unfocused. They try to do too much in any one treatment with needles so the range of their treatments is too wide to be effective. Too many signals are given to the body to clearly redirect energy. By trying to treat every symptom beginners end up treating very little.

Tunnel vision is the opposite of the shotgun approach. This is again the fundamental problem of not seeing the larger picture of the patterns and interrelationships. However, instead of trying to do too much, the practitioner focuses myopically on one thing. For example, the practitioner may always assume that knee problems mean Kidney problems and therefore hone in on only one facet of the case. The balance between these two extremes is the ability to see the pattern of the pathogenesis. Points are chosen for their synergistic effects, that is, for how they work together to treat the pattern of the illness, not just the symptoms.

Point selection must be efficient. Choose points with a multiplicity of functions that will meet the therapeutic aim. Clinical experience seems to bear out that "less is more and more is less," meaning points should be selected that meet the diagnostic criteria. My preference is to use few points and to use only those that are directly related to the treatment plan. Because few points are chosen so as not to confuse the redirecting of the body's energy, points with a multiplicity of energetics are the most efficient.

Again, we choose points for their synergistic effects, that is, for how they work together to treat the whole pattern of illness.

Clinically effective points may be chosen, that is, points with known therapeutic value. Clinically effective points may be points on the fourteen meridians or points that are part of the Extra point system.

In most cases of tonification, needles should be inserted from top to bottom to bring the energy down, in order to root and secure it. For example, when there is too much energy in the head or upper part of the body, points should be selected from the lower part of the body. Infantile convulsion and migraine are effectively treated this way with points such as KI 1 (*Yongquan*) and GB 41 (*Zulinqi*) respectively. However, there are instances in emergency situations such as fainting when the Clear *Qi* does not rise and the treatment points such as GV 26 (*Shuigou*) on the top of the body and HT 9 (*Shaochong*) on the extremities are indicated.

Other treatment directives include first treating the front and then the back; treating the right before the left; and needling from the midline to the lateral side. The theoretical justification for each of these three strategies is to bring *Yin* (front/right/middle) into *Yang* (back/left/lateral). For example, if CV 12 and ST 21 (*Liangmen*) are being needled, needle CV 12 (*Zhongwan*) first and then ST 21 (*Liangmen*). Then, withdraw the needles in the order of insertion.

Needle each point singularly for its unique energetics, for example, SP 6 (*Sanyinjiao*) for edema of the lower limbs.

Needle a chain of points along a meridian or in an affected area to strengthen the therapeutic aim. For example, for Gall Bladder sciatica, needle GB 30 (*Huantiao*), GB 34 (*Yanglingquan*), GB 40 (*Qiuxu*), and GB 44 (*Zuqiaoyin*).

Encircle a point with needles. For example, needling all around the area in a circle of points can treat the navel, which should not be needled directly. Needle specifically eight points 0.5 cun around the navel, called the KI 16 (*Huangshu*) area.

Case 3 offers an example of using a particular treatment strategy to achieve improvement.

CASE 3: THE USE OF DISTAL POINTS FOR KNEE PAIN

The patient was a 45-year-old woman whose major complaint was traumatic arthritis on the medial side of her knee, exacerbated by her occupation as a gardener. She did much of her work on her knees without protection. In addition, she had tendonitis of the arms, calcification of the elbow, and low back pain. Apart from her major complaint, the patient presented with a condition of agitation and stress. Because of monetary concerns, she wanted quick results. She was highly resistant to answering any questions that she felt were not relevant to the major complaint and also insisted that needles be inserted at her knee.

My approach was to ask many of the traditional questions and to do a thorough physical exam to assess the root of the problem. The patient's demand for quick resolution of the problem challenged my ability to determine the root cause of the disease. Finally, because of her uncooperative attitude about the questioning and about the tongue and pulse examinations, I selected palpation of the abdomen and the knee to ascertain etiology. The patient still could not understand why attention was being placed on the abdomen over her knee but I was adamant about this particular procedure.

Needles were placed locally around the knee in the first treatment. However, the emotionally volatile patient clearly reported that she could feel more benefit from the distal points used to rectify abdominal tension, discomfort, or deficiency. After the first treatment, the patient was considerably less demanding and demonstrative and told me to do whatever I thought was necessary. The knee, back, and tendonitis all felt better, and by the fourth treatment the patient effusively thanked me for her relief and vowed she would be back at the slightest sign of aggravation.

Three years later the patient returned for manifestations of stress. The original major complaint of the knee problem that brought her to me was a thing of the past. This is an example of a treatment strategy in which the local area was not the area of choice for treatment. More distal points that affect that area for other reasons corrected the root in fewer than four treatments.

THE TREATMENT OF HEADACHES WITH UNUSUAL CLINICALLY EFFECTIVE POINTS, LOCAL AND DISTAL POINTS

Millions of people endure headaches on a daily basis. While some cope relatively successfully with the pain, mainly with analgesics, for others this pain is an inescapable fact of life. Books on the treatment of disease more than adequately recognize this affliction that characterizes the human condition and suggest various treatment strategies for the different types of headaches that can occur and those books can be consulted. However, there are other useful treatment approaches not found in the classical literature that are based on additional differentiations discussed herein. Table 9.3 lists six common types of headache, their corresponding *Zang-fu* differentiation, and their primary treatment points not found in classical literature.

Table 9.3. The Treatment of Headaches with Unusual
Points Not Found in Classical Literature

Type of Headache	*Zang-Fu* Differentiation	Point Use
Vertical	Liver	CV 12 (*Zhongwan*)
Band type	Spleen *Qi* deficiency with Damp	CV 12 (*Zhongwan*)
Frontal	*Yangming* (ST/LI)	CV 12 (*Zhongwan*)
Behind ears	Triple Burner	CV 12 (*Zhongwan*)
Occipital	Bladder	BL 40 (*Weizhong*)
Temporal	Gall Bladder/Triple Burner	TB 9 (*Sidu*) and GB 36 (*Waiqiu*)

The rationale for using each point is given in Table 9.3 and is well justified, but obviously these are rather uncommon points. The treatment of headache with these unusual points illustrates how important it is to understand the internal pathways of meridians, an understanding that opens up new and clearly effective treatment strategies. As I have discussed in other sections in this book, the major treatment points may be used either alone or as the primary point in a broader treatment plan.

Before using these points, we must decide how to needle them. For instance, for a headache at the vertex, CV 12 (*Zhongwan*) is the recommended point. However, should the point be tonified or dispersed? The answer, of course, depends on the nature of the headache at the vertex. For instance, if the headache has strong pounding pain, it is due to Liver *Yang* rising, so CV 12 (*Zhongwan*) would be dispersed. If there is emptiness or even cold, the headache is from *Blood* deficiency, so CV 12(*Zhongwan*) would be tonified. The same would hold true for differentiating a frontal headache. If the headache is dull and nagging, it could be from *Qi* deficiency, so CV 12 (*Zhongwan*) would be tonified. If there is stuffiness or nausea, the headache could be from food stagnation, so the point would be dispersed. By understanding the different types of pain and the functional spheres of the *Zang-fu* organs, the practitioner can formulate a diagnosis, the treatment plan, and the appropriate needle technique.

Case 4 described here illustrates the combination of local and distal points in treatment.

CASE 4: FOOD POISONING HEADACHE TREATED WITH A COMBINATION OF LOCAL AND DISTAL POINTS

The patient had just arrived at my clinic for a weekly treatment and was experiencing an acute stomachache. She had lunch at a small fast food restaurant with questionable sanitary conditions. She was doubled over in pain, which was spasmodic and colicky. She also had an intense, pounding frontal headache that was making her nauseous.

With the patient in a reclining position, I applied a strong dispersion technique to ST 34 (*Liangqiu*), the *Xi* (cleft) point of the Stomach meridian. Within a few minutes the Stomach pain stopped. However, she still had the headache, so I continued to work on CV 12 (*Zhongwan*), the Influential point that dominates all the *Fu* organs as well as being the Front *Mu* point of the Stomach. Shortly thereafter, the headache and nausea also stopped and the patient was able to leave the office feeling fine.

Summary

As seen herein and in the cases presented, there are rules of point selection that dictate point choice and the order of the insertion of needles. Think about if you use any methodology in your needling strategies and if the ones presented in this chapter make sense to you.

Chapter 10

Written Communications, Patient Plans, and Consent Forms

Learning Objectives

In this brief chapter the importance of consent forms and written communications with patients is discussed. It is highly recommended that you use handouts for your patients, either ones you have devised or the forms I have provided you with that you can modify for your own practice. Written communications should offer patients clear steps to follow for their healthcare and many improve patient compliance in their own treatment. Likewise, you can keep a copy of those directions for your patient files for good recordkeeping. Herein you will learn how to employ them successfully.

When a patient comes for medical treatment it can be a simple, to complicated, to overwhelming experience. Regardless of the quality of the encounter it is imperative that in order to do no harm to the patient as a healthcare provider that the patient clearly understands any instructions that you might offer that you want them to follow. Because some advice for certain conditions may be similar but have some differentiating aspects I highly recommend the use of patient plans. Consent forms are legally required so you must use them. To assist you as a novice to advanced practitioner, I have provided you with several such forms that I have devised and that you are welcome to use and adapt for your own practice. Each is discussed below.

THE CLINICAL REPORT FORM

The Clinical Report From is a document that I devised to accompany the needle technique classes that I teach. Essentially it is a logical methodology that I use to guide the students through the thought processes of intake, to treatment evaluation from start to finish. This form incorporates the exquisite logic of Chinese medicine and how every step from intake to results is documented. This form can also be deconstructed and used in a narrative form once the student becomes a licensed practitioner. While practitioners may feel that they know what they are doing, and most likely they do, reminding ourselves of why in writing, like an outline, should aid us in all of the steps of clinical delivery. After thirty years of using this form as a teacher, every year, the biggest deficiencies that is I see in students are the following, hence the importance of such a form. They are detailed herein.

1. A failure to *differentiate* the major complaint.

2. A failure to provide a rationale or a reason as to why they have selected a particular modality.

3. A failure to justify the use of the acupuncture points selected for treatment apart from points based upon memorized indications without understanding why that indication is called for.

For instance, with a major complaint of tiredness, we should recognize that it could have numerous etiologies. Tiredness alone, by itself, does not give us enough information to arrive at a diagnosis. Is the tiredness due to *Qi* deficiency, *Blood* deficiency, *Yin* deficiency, *Yang* deficiency, or Dampness or any stagnation? Are specific organs involved such as *Qi* deficiencies of the Lung, Spleen, Heart, or Kidney or a combination of several? Is there *Blood* deficiency in general or of the Liver or Heart? Are there any other etiologies? In short, without differentiating the major complaint we cannot arrive at a diagnosis. For instance, the tiredness as the major complaint, accompanied by further symptoms of pallor, shortness of breath, and catching colds easily suggests the diagnosis of Lung *Qi* deficiency. Concomitantly, the treatment plan will be to tonify the Lung *Qi*.

The next question would be how to tonify the Lung *Qi*, that is, with which modality or tool? In many cases the answer will be to select needles, However in instances of tonifying the *Yang*, moxibustion might be a better choice due to the ability of moxa to warm the cold, dry Damp, and penetrate to the meridian level.

The point selection should be related to the diagnosis. For instance, in the previous case a typical student answer is LU 1 (*Zhongfu*) because it is good for Lung problems, LU 5 (*Chize*) because it is good for shortness of breath, or even any point on the Lung meridian! But what makes each point special? What is each point's unique contribution to body physiology? If the diagnosis is Lung *Qi* deficiency, which points combined with a tonification method of the needle can tonify Lung *Qi*? Would BL 13 (*Feifu*) be a good point as the Back *Shu* point of the Lung that affects organ *Qi*? Could it be KI 16 (*Huangshu*), which tonifies the Spleen because Spleen is the mother of Lung and hence nourishes the Lung? Remember the advice of the classics, "When an element is deficient tonify the mother." In this case tonifying earth strengthens metal. Overall the rule of thumb is to choose points based upon categories that they belong to in the point classification system discussed in Chapter 8 versus the memorization of point indications.

Even advanced practitioners can use this short, clear form to document their treatments.

Form 1. The Clinical Report Form

Date of treatment . . . .

Patient age, major complaint (MC) and accompanying differentiating signs and symptoms (AC)

MC . . . .

AC . . . .

Diagnosis (DX) and Treatment Plan (TP)

DX . . . .

TP . . . .

Modality used (i.e. needles, moxa, etc.) and rationale, that is, why is the modality suitable?

. . . .

. . . .

Protocol used if any and rationale

. . . .

. . . .

Treatment (describe in full)

Points used and energetics relevant to treatment plan

. . . .

Type of needle used – gauge, length

. . . .

Method of needling; tonification, dispersion, angle and depth of insertion, etc. and why

. . . .

Bilateral or unilateral treatment and why

. . . .

Retention time and why

. . . .

Moxa or other adjunct therapy in detail

. . . .

Outcome of treatment, how patient felt, etc.

. . . .

. . . .

. . . .

. . . .

PATIENT HANDOUT PLAN

For the most part patients like to be involved in their healthcare management. Having patients do certain things at home such as self-moxa, exercise, following particular dietary guidelines, or massaging acupuncture points can improve health outcomes. Patients may forget what to do and how to follow some directions. Providing them with a written handout or instruction sheet can enhance therapeutic outcomes and assist patients with better following instructions. For this purpose, a patient handout plan, Form 2, has been devised that you might use or modify for your practice.

Form 2. Patient Handout Plan

ABOUT YOUR VISIT

For . . . . Date . . . .

Practitioner . . . .

It was a pleasure to assist you with your healthcare today. I trust that your experience was helpful and I look forward to participating in your future healthcare.

During your visit we discussed

. . . .

. . . .

. . . .

. . . .

. . . .

. . . .

. . . .

Your next appointment has been scheduled for . . . .

Please call if your symptoms do not improve or worsen with this plan of treatment or if you have any questions.

INFORMED CONSENT FOR ACUPUNCTURE

All treatments should be preceded by informed consent for acupuncture. Consent to treatment is important in any medical tradition. Patients have a right to make informed choices. The framework of informed consent seeks to achieve a balance between respecting the patient's autonomy and the physician's highest calling to do good, called beneficence, and doing no harm. Informed consent is not a medical Miranda warning but rather an integrative process whereby the patient's and the physician's thinking become transparent to each other. Consent forms can ensure privacy, confidentiality, but most of all knowledge by which the patient makes an informed choice. Signature on a consent form is only evidence that the patient has signed a piece of paper and this is an important step, however it never replaces explaining any procedure to a patient. Interestingly in the allopathic world the readability of informed consent forms has been shown to exceed the average reading levels of most adults in the United States! How can this mean anything? Consent for treatment must be both verbal and in writing and it is incumbent upon the practitioner to explain any treatment procedure and its benefits, risks, and alternatives.

If you subscribe to medical malpractice insurance, and it is highly recommended that you do so, you will most likely be provided with standardized Consent to Acupuncture Treatment forms that you must use for malpractice purposes. Additionally, those forms will require the patient to agree to arbitration before initiating a lawsuit. If you have malpractice you will need to use their forms, hence a sample is not provided.

The insurance form suffices for any Oriental medical treatment that you might administer, however check your particular policy. Because certain modalities such as moxibustion, fire cupping, and *Gwa Sha* have added risks I have devised special forms for their administration. While they are not needed I find that they heighten my consciousness and explain their unique applications to the patient. Such a form is analogous to any informed consent that a medical doctor would employ although it will have the differentiating aspects that correspond to acupuncture treatment.

INFORMED CONSENT FOR MOXIBUSTION

Moxibustion is the other side of the coin to acupuncture, so much so that the Chinese characters are intertwined as one. As practitioners know, while needles can cause damage if used incorrectly so too can moxibustion. As a result patients need to be informed of the therapeutic benefits of moxa as well as its risks. These outcomes can be found in the Informed Consent for Moxibustion form. Go thorough it verbally with the patient and have them read and sign it.

Form 3. Informed Consent for Moxibustion

INFORMED CONSENT FOR MOXIBUSTION TREATMENT

I request and consent to the performance of the moxibustion treatments, which I have initialed below, on me (or on the patient named for whom I am legally responsible) by the practitioner of Oriental Medicine and/or other practitioners of Oriental medicine who now or in the future treat me while employed by, working or associated with or serving as back-up for the practitioner, including those working at the clinic or office listed whether signatories to this form or not.

I understand that all moxibustion includes the application of heat to acupuncture points and other areas of my body by manipulating a burning herb in various ways, to allow the heat to warm and penetrate my skin. I understand that there are some risks to moxibustion treatment, including but not limited to, a risk of burn and/or scarring. The risk of infection is also present if burning occurs.

Patient's Initials . . . . Date . . . .

I agree to treatment with indirect moxa. I understand that this treatment includes the application of burning moxa near my skin. I understand that this procedure is not intended to result in burns and scarring, but that burning and scarring is a possibility.

Patient's Initials . . . . Date . . . .

I have been instructed to apply indirect moxa to myself. My practitioner has instructed me in this procedure and I understand the instructions. I realize that this procedure includes the application of burning moxa near my skin. I understand that this procedure is not intended to result in burns and scarring, but that burning and scarring is a possibility.

Patient's Initials . . . . Date . . . .

I agree to treatment with direct moxa. I understand that this includes the direct application of burning moxa near my skin and often results in burns and scarring. In fact, burning and scarring may even be part of the therapeutic action, and may be intentional on the part of the practitioner for therapeutic purposes.

Patient's Initials . . . . Date . . . .

I consent to treatment with moxa in any form. Please note this in my chart in the "Medical Alert Section".

Patient's Initials . . . . Date . . . .

In summary

I have had an opportunity to discuss with the practitioner the nature and purpose of this moxibustion treatment. I understand that results are not guaranteed.

I do not expect the practitioner to be able to anticipate and explain all risks and complications. I wish to rely on the practitioner to exercise judgment which the practitioner feels at the time is in my best interest, based upon the facts then known, during the course of the procedure.

I understand that I have the choice to accept or reject the proposed procedure or treatment, or any part of it, before or during the treatment.

I have read, or have had read to me, the consent form. I have also had an opportunity to ask questions about its content, and by signing I agree to the procedures. I intend this consent form to cover the entire course of treatment for my present condition and for any future condition(s) for which I seek treatment.

PATIENT'S SIGNATURE . . . . DATE . . . .
(or patient representative, please indicate relationship to patient)

PRACTITIONER'S SIGNATURE . . . . DATE . . . .

Self-administered moxibustion can assist the patient in more frequent treatment that can contribute to their healthcare. Yet moxibustion is not without its concomitant risks if it is used incorrectly. It is the practitioner's responsibility to instruct the patient on the correct use of any moxa modality including its demonstration. A written consent form, Directions for Self-Treatment at Home with Moxa, has been provided to you for this purpose.

Form 4. Directions for Self-Treatment at Home with Moxa

DIRECTIONS FOR SELF-TREATMENT AT HOME WITH MOXA

Please read all of these instructions through thoroughly before using moxa on yourself.

There are risks involved with moxibustion treatment. The risks include, but are not limited to a burn and/or scarring, and possible infection if burning occurs.

The following procedure is to be followed when applying moxibustion.

1. All patients must be informed of the risks, benefits and alternatives to moxibustion prior to treatment. The practitioner must go over the "Informed Consent for Moxibustion Treatment" form with each patient, prior to instruction for moxa use, or purchase of moxa from this office.

2. All patients must understand and sign the "Informed Consent for Moxibustion Treatment" form prior to treatment, instruction for use, or purchase of moxa from this office.

3. Patients must demonstrate, to the practitioner's satisfaction, the ability to perform moxibustion on him/herself prior to any purchase of moxa in the office.

Patient Instructions:

Using moxa at home

All moxa is to be applied only until your skin becomes mildly pink and/or warm to the touch to achieve the desired level of therapeutic action. Your practitioner will instruct you in this. You must continually monitor the temperature of your skin, to ensure against inadvertent burning. In order to prevent inadvertent burns, do not use moxa on areas that are numb or have any lack of feeling.

If using the moxa pole/stick light one end of the moxa pole with a lighter the way you would light an incense stick. When it is well lit, blow out the flame. It will smoke and when you blow on this end it should glow red at the tip. The tip of the moxa stick is now very hot and could burn you if you are not careful.

Once the moxa stick is lit, bring it to about an inch from the skin for only about one second, and then move it to about six inches above the skin for about two seconds. Repeat this one-second two-second "pecking" motion for about five minutes or until your skin becomes sufficiently red and/or warm as you have been shown.

You must continually monitor the temperature of your skin in order to adjust or remove the moxa pole as necessary.

If at any time your skin should get too hot, remove the moxa stick far from your person.

Avoid the possibility of fire. Moxa poles can be tricky to extinguish so it is recommended that you put a few drops of water on the burning tip of the pole to put it out completely. If you are judicious in the amount of water used the pole should be dry enough to be lit again. If not, you can carefully cut off the damp tip.

Care for Moxa burns:

All moxa burns are to be treated as burns with standard first aid treatment.

Small moxa burns where there is no broken skin are to be kept clean and covered with a sterile dressing. Should any signs of infection develop you are advised to seek emergency medical care from a qualified Western medical professional.

For burns that are severe, large, or break the skin, the patient should immediately seek a qualified Western medical professional for emergency treatment.

Two other popular Chinese medical modalities, *Gwa Sha* and fire cupping, have distinct benefits and some possible side effects. As a result it is preferable to inform the patient in writing of these outcomes. To assist in such communication the following two informed consent forms are offered: Form 5 is Informed Consent for *Gwa Sha* Treatment and Form 6 is Informed Consent for Fire Cupping.

Form 5. Informed Consent for *Gwa Sha* Treatment

I request and consent to the performance of the *Gwa Sha* treatment, which I have initialed below, on me (or on the patient named below, for whom I am legally responsible) by the practitioner.

Gwa Sha Treatment, Risks and Discomforts

Gwa Sha is intended to promote the circulation of *Qi* and *Blood*, which may cause a small amount of blood to arise under the skin surface resulting in a bruise like appearance. There are some discomforts to *Gwa Sha* treatment, including but not limited to large discolorations of the skin that could range from pink, red, or black as well as small reddish dots on the skin. These marks are subcutaneous blemishing, which may take two to four days to fade.

I understand that *Gwa Sha* includes repeated pressured strokes to the skin.

Patient's Initials . . . . Date . . . .

I have had an opportunity to discuss with the practitioner the nature and purpose of this *Gwa Sha* treatment. I understand that results are not guaranteed.

I do not expect the practitioner to be able to anticipate and explain all risks and complications. I wish to rely on the practitioner to exercise judgment which the practitioner feels at the time is in my best interest, based upon the facts then known, during the course of this procedure.

I understand that I have the choice to accept or reject the proposed procedure or treatment, or any part of it, before or during the treatment.

I have read, or have had read to me, the consent form. I have also had an opportunity to ask questions about its content, and by signing I agree to these procedures. I intend this consent form to cover the entire course of treatment for any present condition and for any future condition(s) for which I seek treatment with *Gwa Sha*.

PATIENT'S SIGNATURE . . . . DATE . . . .
(or patient representative, please indicate relationship to patient)

PRACTITIONER'S SIGNATURE . . . . DATE . . . .

Form 6. Informed Consent for Fire Cupping

I request and consent to the performance of Fire Cupping treatment, which I have initialed below, on me by the practitioner named below and/or other practitioners of Oriental medicine who now or in the future treat me while employed by, working or associated with, or serving as back up for the practitioner named below, including those working at the clinic or office listed below, whether signatories to this form or not.

There are some risks to fire cupping treatments, including but not limited to a risk of burn and/or scarring, and blisters of the skin around cups. The risk of infection is also present if burning occurs.

I understand that all fire cupping includes the usage of cups, alcohol, and fire to create a negative pressure on the skin over acupuncture points, and other areas of my body. By manipulating a cup it allows the suction to promote circulation of *Qi* and *Blood* to the area being treated.

Patient's Initials . . . .   Date . . . .

I agree to treatment with fire cups. I understand that this treatment includes the application of cups to areas of my body with the use of glass cups, alcohol, and fire. I understand this procedure is not intended to result in burns and blisters, but that burning and blistering of the skin around the cups is a possibility.

Patient's Initials . . . .   Date . . . .

I have had the opportunity to discuss with the practitioner named below the nature and purpose of this fire cupping treatment. I do not expect the practitioner to be able to anticipate and explain all risks and complications. I wish to rely on the practitioner to exercise judgment which the practitioner judges at the time is in my best interest, based upon the facts then known, during the course of this procedure. I understand that I have the choice to accept or reject the proposed procedure or treatment, or any part of it, before or during treatment.

I have read, or have had read to me, the consent form. I have also had an opportunity to ask questions about its content, and by signing below I agree to the procedure. I intend this consent form to cover the entire course of treatment for my present condition and for any future condition(s) for which I seek treatment.

PATIENT'S SIGNATURE . . . . DATE . . . .
(or patient representative, please indicate relationship to patient)

PRACTITIONER'S SIGNATURE . . . . DATE . . . .

I have discussed the above information with the patient, including the risks, benefits, and alternatives to the proposed treatment.

PRACTITIONER'S SIGNATURE . . . . DATE . . . .

Summary

The importance of informed consent cannot be over estimated legally or ethically. These forms further build rapport by improving communication and the understanding of the patient's own healthcare.

Chapter 11

Acupuncture Emergencies

Learning Objectives

The best way to manage needle shock and acupuncture accidents such as fainting or lightheadedness is to avoid them in the first place. This can be achieved through proper needling and attention to the patient's condition. However, if they do occur you need to have an appropriate first response. For clinician convenience that information is summarized in this chapter in an outline form that can be posted on a bulletin board in your treatment room or office for quick consultation.

NEEDLE SHOCK AND MANAGING ACCIDENTS
1. Prevention

- Do not treat patients who are too weak, too tired, or too hungry

- Do not treat patients who have eaten too much, appear intoxicated, or are on mind altering drugs including alcohol

- Correctly position the patient for needling

- Do not needle too forcefully, too deeply, for too long, or with too many needles

2. Signs of acupuncture sickness

- Pallor

- Shallow or rapid breathing

- Unconsciousness or fainting

- Sweaty hands, face, chest, or feet

- Lightheadedness

- Increased or decreased body temperature

3. If signs of needle shock/acupuncture sickness develop

- Stay calm

- Withdraw all the needles

- Elevate the feet

- Cover the torso with a blanket

- Press on resuscitation points

- GV 26 (*Renzhong*) will bring the energy up to the head if the patient is dizzy or lightheaded

- KI 1 (*Yongquan*) will bring the energy down if the person is nervous, anxious, or needs to be grounded

- In severe cases, in addition to the above management, press hard with your thumb or needle PC 9 (*Zhongchong*), GV 25 (*Suliao*) PC 6 (*Neiguan*), ST 36 (*Zusanli*), or CV 4 (*Guanyuan*)

- Generally the patient will respond to these measures but if not, other emergency steps should be taken such as calling 911

- Administer a warm drink *if* conscious

- If you know that the person is diabetic, hypoglycemic, or hungry, and they are weak after they have recovered, offer juice, sweetened drinks, crackers, or a small carbohydrate such as a cookie or candy. Always make sure to have some such food or drink on hand

Chapter 12

Ten Needle Technique

Learning Objectives

Ten Needle Technique is a powerful treatment strategy that tonifies the foundational energy of the body, the subject of this book. Though the use of these classical Chinese acupoints the root energy of the body can be accessed and strengthened, helping in the treatment of unlimited diseases that can be differentiated in broad paradigmatic terms. Ten Needle Technique is an elegant, time-tested clinical strategy that can be used repeatedly week to week to strengthen the baseline energy of the body.

In chronic conditions, when deficiency of *Qi*, *Blood*, or *Yin* is the primary diagnosis, Ten Needle Technique treatment can be used as either a treatment strategy in and of itself or as a skeletal formula to which other points are added based upon signs and symptoms. This treatment is effective in tonifying *Yang* as well especially when moxa is applied to applicable points such as ST 36 (*Zusanli*) or on the abdomen. This formula can be applied in a variety of clinical situations. It is obvious in clinical practice that deficiency of the essential substances of *Qi*, *Blood*, *Yin*, and *Yang* are not only commonly encountered but may be considered difficult to treat because they indicate long-term, chronic conditions. Thus, this formula, which can tonify *Qi*, *Blood*, *Yin*, and *Yang*, is certainly an efficient prescription.

A discussion of the primary energetics that account for the utility of this valuable formula follows. A note of caution should be observed concerning the insertion depths of these needles, which are the recommended depths from Chinese texts. As always, these depths are a range and should be adjusted according to the patient's presentation. For instance, many patients are thin, guarded, or vulnerable in the abdominal region and along the Conception Vessel channel so the more shallow depths of insertion may be indicated. Table 12.1 summarizes the points used in Ten Needle Technique, their locations, angles, and insertion depths.

Table 12.1. Ten Needle Technique: Points, Locations, Angles, and Depths of Insertions

Points	Locations	Angles and Depths of Insertions
CV 13 (*Shangguan*)	On the midline of the abdomen, 5 *cun* above the center of the umbilicus	Perpendicular .5 in.–1.2 in.
CV 12 (*Zhongwan*)	On the midline of the abdomen, 4 *cun* above the center of the umbilicus	Perpendicular .5 in.–1.2 in.
CV 10 (*Xiawan*)	On the midline of the abdomen, 2 *cun* above the center of the umbilicus	Perpendicular .5 in–1.2 in.
ST 25 (*Tianshu*) (bilateral)	2 *cun* lateral to the center of the umbilicus	Perpendicular .7 in–1.2 in. The moxa box can be added from CV 10 (*Xiawan*) to ST 25 (*Tianshu*) and below to tonify *Yang*
ST 36 (*Zusanli*) (bilateral)	3 *cun* below ST 35 (*Dubi*), 1 finger breadth lateral to the anterior crest of the tibia	Perpendicular .5 in–1.2 in.
CV 6 (*Qihai*)	On the midline of the abdomen, 1.5 *cun* below the umbilicus	Perpendicular .8 in.–1.2 in.
PC 6 (*Neiguan*) (bilateral)	2 *cun* above the wrist crease, between the tendons of the muscles palmaris longus and flexor carpi radialis	Perpendicular .5 in–.8 in.

CLINICAL ENERGETICS OF THE POINTS
CV 13 (*Shangguan*)

This point controls the upper orifice of the Stomach, the cardiac sphincter, so that food can enter the Stomach to begin the rottening and ripening process. In this way the Stomach *Qi* descends more fully to continue the digestive process to produce *Qi*, *Blood*, and *Yin*.

CV 12 (*Zhongwan*)

CV 12 (*Zhongwan*) combined with CV 13 (*Shangguan*) raises the *Yang* and sinking Spleen *Qi*. CV 12 (*Zhongwan*), the Front *Mu* point of the Stomach, is one of the Eight Influential points that dominate the *Fu* organs. As such, it is involved in receiving and digesting, excreting food. It regulates Stomach *Qi* and tonifies chronic Spleen and Stomach problems such as deficiency of *Qi*, *Yin*, or *Yang*. It also resolves Dampness. CV 12 (*Zhongwan*) is a very powerful point as an important vortex or Crossing point of many meridians. The following energies center around it:

- The internal pathway of the Lung meridian begins at CV 12 (*Zhongwan*).

- The Spleen, Heart, and Small Intestine meridians pass through CV 12 (*Zhongwan*).

- The Liver meridian ends there.

- The Large Intestine and Triple Burner meridians begin there.

- The point is located along the Conception Vessel channel pathway.

- Located at the midpoint of the Stomach, the point controls the middle of the Stomach, tonifying the Spleen and Stomach so they can produce *Qi*, *Blood*, and *Yin* and resolve Dampness. It regulates Stomach *Qi* and is useful for chronic Stomach and Spleen problems. It suppresses rebellious Stomach *Qi* and is good for neurasthenia and emotional problems.

CV 10 (*Xiawan*)

Xiawan controls the lower orifice of the Stomach, the pylorus, encouraging Stomach *Qi* to descend. It relieves food stagnation and tonifies the Spleen and Stomach so that food is broken down and transformed into *Qi*, *Blood*, or *Yin*. Because of its lower location in relation to the Stomach, it is helpful in resolving indigestion, stomachache, and prolapse of the Stomach, diarrhea, and acute Stomach problems.

ST 25 (*Tianshu*)

As the Front *Mu* point of the Large Intestine, according to the *Neijing* (*The Yellow Emperor's Classic*), ST 25 (*Tianshu*) adjusts the intestines in any condition, that is, it clears heat, regulates *Qi*, relieves food retention, and eliminates stagnation.

According to the *Nanjing* (*The Classic of Difficult Questions*), Stomach 25 (*Tianshu*) is the Front *Mu* point of the Lungs, hence the condition of the Lungs can be determined at ST 25 (*Tianshu*) on the right side of the body. According to Yoshio Manaka, ST 25 (*Tianshu*) is the Front *Mu* point of the Triple Burner on the right side of the body

On the left side ST 25 (*Tianshu*) is an extremely reliable indicator of *Blood* stagnation and Liver *Blood* stagnation in particular. The reason for this is that at ST 25 (*Tianshu*) on the left the portal vein, the only vein that comes off of the Large Intestine, carries nutrients to the Liver to be packaged into packets of glycogen or stored energy. As a result, when Liver *Qi* is stagnant, it frequently leads to Liver *Blood* stagnation and manifests at ST 25 (*Tianshu*) on the left because of this Liver–Large Intestine connection. Correspondingly, when there is a blockage at Stomach 25 (*Tianshu*) on the left, it can cause Liver *Qi* stagnation. When this point is not blocked and is freeflowing, it opens the Lower Burner (*Jiao*) and the channels to nourish the *Qi* of the lower *Jiao*. As such it is a storehouse of energy.

ST 36 (*Zusanli*)

ST 36 (*Zusanli*) opens the Lower Burner, regulates the intestines, and builds Kidney *Yin*. It brings energy down. It benefits and regulates the Stomach and Spleen, controlling the epigastric area. As the Lower *He* (Sea) point, ST 36

(*Zusanli*) sends a vessel directly to the Stomach. As the Horary point on an earth meridian, ST 36 (*Zusanli*) tonifies and balances the *Qi* and *Blood* of the whole body. It stimulates *Qi* production and dispels cold. It strengthens the body's resistance, increases immunity, and strengthens the antipathogenic factor. It regulates *Yin* and *Wei Qi*. It raises the *Yang* and strengthens weak and deficient conditions.

CV 6 (*Qihai*)

This point is at the center of the vital energy in the body, the *Dan Tian*, where the living *Qi* of the Kidney resides. It is useful for all states of exhaustion and insufficiency. Especially with the use of moxa, it tonifies *Qi*, *Yang*, and *Yin*; regulates Qi, tonifies original *Qi*, resolves Damp, augments Kidney deficiency, and strengthens the will to live.

PC 6 (*Neiguan*)

PC 6 (*Neiguan*) assists in communication between and treatment of the three *Jiaos*; it keeps *Qi* and *Blood* flowing in their proper pathways if they are rebellious. As Master of the *Yinwei Mai*, it produces *Yin* defensive energy. Coupled with the Spleen meridian and the *Chong Mai* vessel, PC 6 (*Neiguan*) assists Spleen and Kidney functions.

In accordance with rules of point insertion, insert needles from top to bottom, right to left, and medial to lateral. Note the Pericardium is the first point to needle as it is in the Upper *Jiao* according to Chinese anatomical positioning. The exception here is to needle Stomach 25 (*Tianshu*) on the left first to unblock any stagnation at that point since it connects to the Liver via the portal vein. It also unblocks any stagnation at the junction of the transverse and descending colons.

APPLICATIONS

An example of using Ten Needle Technique in combination with other points would be to add CV 3 (*Zhongji*), Front *Mu* point of the Bladder, and SP 6 (*Sanyinjiao*), Group *Luo* of the Three Leg *Yin*, for cases of urinary retention. Add moxa for greater therapeutic results as long as there are no signs of heat.

It is apparent from an analysis of the formula that Ten Needle Technique is a beneficial formula to employ when there are many symptoms pointing in the direction of deficiency. But sometimes very deficient patients whom this formula would benefit cannot tolerate the insertion of ten needles, in which case the following modifications can be made:

- Needle PC 6 (*Neiguan*) only on the left side because Pericardium energetics are more left-sided.

- Pretest by palpating CV 13 (*Shangguan*), CV 12 (*Zhongwan*), and CV 10 (*Xiawan*) and select the most deficient point to needle.

- As "Heaven's Pivot," ST 25 (*Tianshu*) should always be needled bilaterally to establish equilibrium between *Qi* and *Blood*. As discussed previously under the energetics of that point, ST 25 (*Tianshu*) on the right side is a *Qi* reflex point and ST 25 (*Tianshu*) on the left is a *Blood* stagnation point. Needling both points helps to balance *Qi* and *Blood*.

- CV 6 (*Qihai*) should always be included in this strategy.

- ST 36 (*Zusanli*) can be needled only on the right side due to the affinity of Stomach energetics for the right.

These modifications can be effective especially if the practitioner's tonification needle technique is proficient enough to compensate for the reduced number of needles.

If no signs of heat are present (either of the excess or deficient type) the addition of your choice of moxa is incomparable, particularly for tonifying the *Yang*. The moxa box is particularly valuable due to its large size. Carefully position the moxa box over the lower abdomen with the upper border of the box just above the navel, close to the CV 10 (*Xiawan*)–CV 9 (*Shuifen*) area. The lower border should be on the abdomen so that it covers CV 6 (*Qihai*) and ST 25 (*Tianshu*) as well. Ignite two three-inch pieces of moxa stick at both ends and allow them to burn for ten to twenty minutes. Exercise caution with patients who have neurological disorders that produce a lack of sensitivity to pain, elderly patients, others with delicate skin, or those who have not had their abdomen and especially the navel recently exposed to sun, or if their navel is an "outie." The first time the box is used, the retention time should be short until the practitioner is sure that the patient can tolerate the heat. Always monitor the heat by checking the patient's skin under the box at periodic intervals.

After the administration of the Ten Needle Technique, patients generally will not experience a great surge of energy, but rather a deep-seated feeling of relaxation and perhaps even tiredness as the energy being tonified consolidates itself on a very deep level. Patients should be advised of this therapeutic reaction so they know what to expect. See Table 12.2 for common systemic, foundational results of using Ten Needle Technique.

Table 12.2. Ten Needle Treatment Results

Relaxed	Stabilized	Centered	Quiet, calmer
Grounded	Reduced anxiety	Deep rejuvenation	Increase in deeper energy
Immediate improvement in digestion and energy after large lunch	*Pain increased, tears	Grounded, more relaxed	No insomnia
*Groggy	Deeply relaxed	Energized, clear headed, food difficulties reduced	Strong, decreased back pain
Relaxed, mentally aware	Energized, clear headed, calm, better appetite and digestion	Relaxed, sore throat gone	Grounded, more relaxed
Able to bear stress	On cloud nine, energized, calm, better appetite, no insomnia for 3–5 days, back is better	Energized, warm	Back pain reduced

(continued)

Relaxed	Stabilized	Centered	Quiet, calmer
Warm to the core	*Spacey	Deep-seated feeling of well being, supported at deep level	Wonderful, great
Enjoyed	Voice stronger	Rested	Comforted
Felt whole, connected	Clean	Less groggy	Stomach warm
*Bit spacey but alert			

* May have been too many needles for the patient or in the case of increase pain there might have been a problem with the needle technique

Summary

Ten Needle Technique is a powerful treatment strategy that treats the foundational energy of the person. Ten Needle Technique can be administered as a course of treatment, that is ten consecutive treatments, or as a periodic tonification treatment. It is one of my favorite protocols. Case 5 describes a rather interesting clinical application of this treatment protocol in the treatment of emotions.

CASE 5: THE APPLICATION OF TEN NEEDLE TECHNIQUE IN THE TREATMENT OF EMOTIONS

The patient was a thirty-five-year-old female with no real physical complaint. She had made an appointment with me for "a tune-up." As a victim of incest, her most long-standing problem was mastering her emotions. She also had lots of stress at work, and she was very high-strung.

In answer to the Ten Questions, the subpathologies included gas, over-thinking, waking up at night, a heavy period, abdominal distention, feeling hot, ravenous appetite, some facial breakouts, feeling tight in the intestines, hip joint pain, nighttime urination, exhaustion from time to time, pinpoint pain in the heart, and occasional vaginal discharge.

She had no Western medical diagnosis and she was taking no medication or treatment for these symptoms that she did not view as significant or problematic. The tongue was reddish-purple, with a red tip and small *Yin* deficiency cracks developing. The surface was rough and had no coating except for a greasy one in the lower *Jiao*. The pulse on the left side was thin and weak in all positions. On the right it was stronger but more superficial and slippery. The most significant palpatory finding was a shallow, tight, hard Stomach at CV 12 (*Zhongwan*).

Fifteen treatments constituted the course of therapy needed for both the practitioner and the patient to feel that she was balanced. At that point, every subpathology listed above was resolved and the patient felt better emotionally. She wanted to be balanced and wanted to learn how to deal with her emotions better. She relied upon the practitioner to educate her about the subpathologies and their significance. When CV 12 (*Zhongwan*), the Front *Mu* of the Stomach, the source of all *Yin*, was no longer tender, the patient reported feeling warm, nurtured, and taken care of. Prior to one of the last treatments, she had an abnormal uterine bleeding at ovulation after which she felt a "new freedom in her abdomen."

The Ten Needle Technique, preceded by abdominal clearing, a Japanese technique, was the primary modality employed, and herbs were also prescribed to supplement the treatment. The patient was very receptive to deep breathing, awareness of body energetics, patient education, and compliance with herbs. She felt that all these modalities had given her the tools to cope better with stress or other problems.

Chapter 13

Eight Needle Technique

Learning Objectives ———————————

In this chapter, another foundational treatment is presented which has great clinical efficacy in the treatment of low back pain. While it is most known for the treatment of back pain, it has powerful systemic effects in tonifying the pre- and postnatal *Qi* of the Kidney.

Back pain is part of the human condition. From any therapeutic perspective, this problem can be understood as the result of the trauma and stress to which the back is normally subject, and the treatment of low back pain is one of the chief complaints for which practitioners are consulted. This condition can be difficult to resolve because of its numerous causes, and the complex anatomy of the human back, but if the diagnosis is correct, successful treatment is possible. From a Chinese perspective, back pain has a close but not exclusive functional relationship to the Kidney, the source of life, and hence such a disorder can serve as a reflection of the vitality of the Kidney, the Gate of Life.

In the case of low back pain from deficiency of Kidney *Qi* and *Yang*, Eight Needle Technique is particularly effective. Because this is their only experience, the doctors with whom I studied in China maintained that Chinese needles must be employed in this treatment strategy to most effectively nourish the Kidney energy and circulate the *Qi* and *Blood*. However, it has been my and my students' experience on hundreds of patients that Japanese needles, even #1 Seirins, can achieve therapeutic results although a #3 or #5 may be better due to the thick musculature of the lower back. Table 13.1 lists the points used in Eight Needle Technique, their corresponding angles, and depths of needle insertion.

Following the table, the primary energetics that contribute to making this formula effective in the treatment of low back pain due to Kidney *Qi* and *Yang* deficiency are discussed.

Table 13.1. Eight Needle Technique: Points, Locations, and Angles and Depths of Insertion

Points	Locations	Angles and Depths of Insertion
BL 23 (*Shenshu*) (bilateral)	1.5 *cun* lateral to the lower border of the spinous process of the 2nd lumbar vertebra	Perpendicular .8 in.–1 in.
GV 4 (*Mingmen*)	In the depression below the lower border of the spinous process of the 2nd lumbar vertebra	Perpendicular .5 in.–1 in. Moxa needle or the moxa box may also be applied here
BL 25 (*Dachangshu*) (bilateral)	1.5 *cun* lateral to the lower border of the spinous process of the 4th lumbar vertebra	Perpendicular .8 in.–1.5 in.
GV 3 (*Yaoyangguan*)	In the depression below the spinous process of the 4th lumbar vertebra level with the iliac crest	Perpendicular .5 in.–1 in.
BL 40 (*Weizhong*) (bilateral)	At the popliteal crease of the knee between the tendons of the muscles biceps femoris and semitendinosus	Perpendicular .5 in.–1.5 in. or bleed No moxa

Note that many of the energetics delineated here pertain to symptoms of Kidney *Qi* and *Yang* deficiency and as such are not limited to the manifestation of low back pain. Consequently, by treating Kidney *Qi* and *Yang* deficiency through these points, there are many added benefits in addition to alleviating low back pain. This formula can also be modified if back pain is not the major complaint, for example, by eliminating BL 40 (*Weizhong*), so as to strengthen the *Qi* of the Kidney. This treatment in turn will benefit many of the domains belonging to Kidney function in Oriental medicine.

CLINICAL ENERGETICS OF THE EIGHT NEEDLE TECHNIQUE POINTS
BL 23 (*Shenshu*)

As the Back *Shu* point of Kidney, BL 23 (*Shenshu*) tonifies and regulates the *Qi* of the Kidney. It is good for strengthening the Kidney's reception of *Qi* in cases of chronic asthma, and benefits the ears in tinnitus or deafness. It is good for chronic eye disorders such as blurred vision, prolapse of the Kidney, weak legs, and irregular menses. It resolves Dampness in the Lower Burner and strengthens the lower back.

Bladder 23 (*Shenshu*) is better for tonifying the *Yang* aspect of Kidney *Qi*, but it can also be used for Kidney *Yin* deficiency. Consequently, it can be used for *Yang* pathologies such as lack of sexual desire, lack of will power, negativity, lack of initiative, depression, dizziness, poor memory, blurred vision, fatigue, constant desire to sleep, cold knees, renal colic, and nephritis. *Yin* deficiencies that it can treat include tidal fever, seizures, and infantile paralysis.

BL 23 (*Shenshu*) nourishes Kidney essence making the point useful in impotence, nocturnal emissions, infertility, and spermatorrhea. It benefits the bones and marrow and is good for any bone pathology. Because it nourishes the *Blood*, it can be used for anemia, brightening the eyes, and alopecia.

GV 4 (*Mingmen*)

The Gate of Life, GV 4 (*Mingmen*), encompasses Kidney *Yin* and *Yang*, which are inextricably bound together. Therefore, GV 4 (*Mingmen*) is appropriate for the two aspects of Kidney *Qi* deficiency, that is, Kidney *Yin* and *Yang*. *Mingmen* tonifies the original *Qi* of the Kidney. In this capacity it nourishes the original *Qi* of pre-heaven, which is the person's constitution, basic vitality, and genetic inheritance on a physical and mental level.

Mingmen is a powerful point to strengthen Kidney *Yang* and all the *Yang* in general, especially if combined with moxa. It tonifies and warms the Fire of the Gate of Vitality, resolving Kidney *Yang* deficiency symptoms such as chilliness, abundant clear urination, diarrhea, and urinary incontinence. *Mingmen* fortifies a tired condition and lack of vitality. It alleviates depression, weak knees, and weak legs. It may be indicated by a pale tongue and a deep, weak pulse. The Japanese call it the essential allergy point, meaning it strengthens the antipathogenic factor.

Mingmen benefits the *Yang* aspect of the Kidney essence and is indicated in all sexual disorders from weakness of essence evidenced by impotence, premature ejaculation, nocturnal emission, and bone disorders. It strengthens the low back and knees, expels cold, and dries Damp-cold, especially with the use of moxa. However, we need to be careful because moxa is very warming and can cause heat aggravation, particularly if there are also signs of Kidney *Yin* deficiency. Discontinue moxa if signs of heat aggravation develop. Other conditions that can be treated include leukorrhea, diarrhea, profuse clear urination, abdominal and uterine pain. *Mingmen* calms the spirit, and benefits and clears the brain. It treats seizures, mania, meningitis, disorientation, forgetfulness, fear, fright, insomnia, and dizziness.

BL 25 (*Dachangshu*)

Dachangshu, BL 25, is the Back *Shu* point of the Large Intestine. Remembering the clinical utility of Back *Shu* points, which are indicated to adjust *Qi* and *Blood*, BL 25 (*Dachangshu*) eliminates stagnation of *Qi* and *Blood* of the intestines that may cause pain, numbness, muscular atrophy, and motor impairment of the back and lower extremities. *Dachangshu* promotes the function of the Large Intestine and removes obstructions from the channel. It regulates the Large Intestine and Stomach, reducing constipation or diarrhea, dysentery, painful defecation or urination, abdominal distention, and intestinal noise. It benefits low back pain or strain, and pain in the sacroiliac joint, and relieves fullness, swelling, and paralysis of the lower extremities. It is the site of most herniated discs.

GV 3 (*Yaoyangguan*)

Yaoyangguan, GV 3, tonifies Kidney *Yang* and *Qi*. As such, it strengthens the lower back and legs. It is beneficial for irregular menstruation, nocturnal emission, and impotence. Very frequently used as a local point for backaches, particularly from Kidney *Yang* deficiency, it is indicated especially when the backache radiates to the legs. It is beneficial for pain in the lumbosacral region, numbness, muscular atrophy, motor impairment, weakness of the legs, and knee pain caused by Kidney *Qi* and *Yang* deficiency. With moxa it warms cold and dries Damp-cold that may produce leukorrhea, diarrhea, colitis, and lower abdominal distention.

BL 40 (*Weizhong*)

Bladder 40 (*Weizhong*) is the *He* (sea) point of the Bladder channel and the Command point of the back. Elementally, it is the earth point and the controlling point of that channel. As such, it is very effective in clearing and resolving heat and Dampness from the Bladder and Intestines that causes burning urination, ulcerations, diarrhea, and urinary incontinence. It clears summer heat in acute attacks of heat in the summertime that manifest as burning fever, delirium, skin rashes, and unconsciousness from heat stroke. It cools the *Blood* and drains heat from the *Blood* especially with bloodletting techniques. Thus, it clears skin diseases, carbuncles, boils, herpes, fever, malarial disorders, restless fetus disorders, and epistaxis.

BL 40 (*Weizhong*) eliminates Blood stasis and channel obstructions that create lower leg or abdominal pain. BL 40 (*Weizhong*) relaxes the sinews and tendons, opens the channel to benefit the lower back, knees, hips, and legs. Although the use of this point is very good for chronic or acute, excess or deficiency type backaches, it is most effective for acute and excess varieties, especially when the backache is either bilateral or unilateral, not on the midline. Lower back pain, sciatica, hip joint pain, restricted movement, lower extremity paralysis, all knee joint diseases, gastrocnemius muscle spasms, convulsions, and muscular tetany can be treated through this point.

As in all cases of tonification and dispersion, needle retention times are relative and will vary. As a general rule, however, needles should be retained for approximately twenty minutes. The needle retention is able to strengthen and deepen the stimulation of the techniques to give greatest effect. Although the overall effect of the treatment is tonification of Kidney *Qi* and *Yang*, the technique applied to each set of points depends on whether the point needs to be tonified or dispersed.

This decision can be made by properly discerning the pathology of each point.

Summary

In conclusion, if the practitioner has secured the correct differentiation of the back pain so that it matches the criteria of Eight Needle Technique, results are swift, efficacious, and long lasting, often with added benefits from tonifying Kidney *Qi* and *Yang* deficiency. See Table 13.2 for common results of the Eight Needle Protocol. Case 6 offers a clinical example of the effectiveness of Eight Needle Technique.

Table 13.2. Eight Needle Treatment Results

Excellent when treatment matches diagnosis
More movement in legs, limber, calmer, centered
Stiff neck better, looser
Warm in low back, warmer in general
More relaxed, rid of stress, relaxed yet energized, invigorated, less muscle tension
Taller, like my back got longer
Pain relief
*Spacey, no improvement, very warm
Better immediately, less pain immediately
Loved it
Energized deeply
Breath deepened
Instantaneous and enormous relief
Coldness reduced, 20–80% improvement
Increased range of motion in hips, relaxed and energized, complexion brighter
Relaxed and lightweight, energized yet peaceful
Back better, legs felt more open
Lighter, relaxed, less tired

Complete relief of back pain, knees and legs felt stronger
Back pain completely gone immediately and for a week follow-up
I could stay here all day
Low back felt better
Sleepy and wanted to go to bed, felt better, more vitality

* Too much moxa used

CASE 6: EIGHT NEEDLE TECHNIQUE FOR BACK PAIN AND OVERALL TONIFICATION

The patient was a thirty-five-year-old woman with a history of chronic lower back problems due to trauma. She also had many signs and symptoms of Kidney *Qi* and *Yang* deficiency such as cold hands and feet, lethargy, problems with memory and concentration, weak legs, blurred vision, irregular, scanty menses, and dizziness. She had received acupuncture for this problem and experienced good to fair results. Scalp acupuncture in particular helped her significantly.

She received an Eight Needle treatment by a student practitioner just learning the technique. The point locations should have been more accurate and the depths of needle insertions should have been deeper. Though the *Qi* was grasped, the tonification technique was weak. In spite of these areas that could have been improved, the patient still reported that during the treatment her back pain diminished. Several days later her back still felt good, though not perfect. However, she was pleasantly surprised to find that in general she felt better, more energetic, and more alert. Her legs were stronger, her eyes brighter, and her head felt less empty. This is a good example of the local and systemic effects of Eight Needle Technique.

Chapter 14

Intradermals

Learning Objectives ————————

The small, short, thin needles, called intradermal needles, are an excellent choice for reinforcing a treatment in the ear or the body. While not specifically a tonification technique per se, these needles are often used in this way. Here the practitioner can reacquaint him or herself in the use of intradermal needles as an adjunct to treatment.

Intradermals are a Japanese adaptation of the classic Chinese through and through or collective loci treatment commonly referred to as threading. In this manner a point may be connected to any other point or stimulated itself by horizontal superficial positioning of the needle in the point in contrast to a perpendicular or oblique insertion.

Intradermals are small subcutaneous needles used to implant an acupoint to promote the same effects as needling but on a sustained basis. They reinforce the action of the point because they are retained. They come in various lengths, most popular being 3mm and 6mm, with 3 being the shortest. The short needles are most often use in the ear, for instance, to thread spinal vertebrae points. Tweezers are used to pick up the intradermal and insert it subcutaneously. The longer intradermals are used on the body such as KI 6 (*Zhaohai*) or SI 3 (*Houxi*). Think about your use of a point and treatment plan to determine if intradermals are a suitable modality. Also consult journal articles or texts on through and through needling.

The most common points selected for treatment are limited but efficacious. They include but are not limited to the following as my favorite points to thread:

- LU 7 (*Lieque*)

- LI 20 (*Yingxiang*) threaded to *Bitong* (Extra point)

- HT 7 (*Shenmen*)

- SI 3 (*Houxi*)

- PC 7 (*Daling*)

- GB 41 (*Zulinqi*)

- *Yintang* (Extra point)

- Wrinkles on the face

These are common points that can be used with intradermals in the ear:

- Adrenal point

- The constipation area

- The spinal segments

- Any grooves such as Frank's sign, the lower blood pressure groove, or tinnitus groove

Practitioners can use their own judgment on the applicability of a point.

Intradermals may be used on the patient in the office in lieu of a needle or retained for take home treatment. If the latter is employed, guard against infection by retaining the intradermals for approximately three to five days depending upon humidity levels or exposure to water. If used in the ear a shower cap should be used or a cotton ball carefully placed in the ear. Provide the patient with written instructions on how to remove them with a tweezer and in what direction to pull out, or to return to your office for removal so that infection does not ensue.

Summary

Intradermal needles are easy to use and efficacious. Carefully use them in treatment as part of your therapeutic tools.

CLINICAL ADAPTATION: FROWN SYNDROME

The area between the eyebrows, known as the glabella in Western anatomical terminology, is a muscular area prone to wrinkles, in some cases very deep ones. In Chinese medicine, in regard to physiognomy, that area represents the Liver. It is the function of the Liver to keep all the energy in the body moving, somewhat akin to *Blood* circulation, as the Liver plays a role in the availability of *Blood* flow in the body. When Liver energy becomes slow or blocked, we call it stagnant. The Liver is the organ in the body most prone to stagnant energy or stagnant *Qi* and *Blood* because it is the organ that moves *Qi* and *Blood*.

Depression in Chinese medicine is defined as Stagnant Liver *Qi*. Hence, if the person has a fair degree of Stagnant Liver *Qi* physiologically, it can become manifest anatomically on the face in the glabella region. The deeper the line or groove, the more Stagnant Liver *Qi* the person is likely to have.

In Oriental medicine there are acupuncture points on the body surface and the underlying superficial muscles in which energy can be accessed and regulated with acupuncture needles. The glabella region encompasses a point called *Yintang*. *Yintang* is a non-meridial point meaning it is not located per se on an energy pathway or one of the fourteen main meridians but in a special place. Such points are called Extra points.

Yintang, located between the medial ends of the two eyebrows, is a relatively large area like an oval. In acupuncture we can needle it subcutaneously downward 0.3–1.0 of an inch and retain it from 5–20 minutes. *Yintang* can also be treated with intradermals either individually for a short wrinkle or in a piggyback fashion for longer ones. "Connect" them by inserting several back to back in a proximal direction towards the nose.

Here is an interesting clinical adaptation to the needling of *Yintang*.

Anatomically, *Yintang* is located above the pituitary gland. Deep and posterior to the pituitary gland at its base is the pineal gland that responds to light and seasonal changes. When light levels are low, the pineal gland secretes melatonin, a hormone that it also manufactures, which is involved in the regulation of sleep and mood disorders. Melatonin has the effect of sedating and relaxing the body, promoting sleep, and improving mood. As such, it is a primary acupuncture point used for these purposes. Patients who have *Yintang* needled frequently return and ask for it to be needled again because of these desired effects. Patients oftentimes refer to it as the "heaven" point because of this pleasant reaction.

Likewise *Yintang* becomes a primary point to treat Seasonal Affective Disorder (SAD), a condition whose primary clinical manifestations are depression and accompanying lethargy. *Yintang* can also be used to treat memory and concentration problems, sinus infections, rhinitis, headache, dizziness, hypertension, and hormonal problems.

Sometimes a reddish coloration is observable at *Yintang*. This red in Oriental medicine indicates heat in the *Blood*, meaning the *Blood* is stagnant and pooling and thus the *Blood* stagnation is observable through the skin. Such a coloration is abnormal, infrequent, and serious, however treatable with conventional acupuncture needling.

Interestingly, when Botox is applied in this area for wrinkles patients miraculously report an improvement in mood and depression. While Botox works to de-innervate the muscle and thus inhibits the contraction of muscles that cause the wrinkle, the needle insertion activates the underlying physiological energetics of the *Yintang* point. This mechanism is akin to the way acupuncture point injection therapy works such as a saline solution or Vitamin B12, that is, injection fluid or the needle simultaneously stimulate the point. Mood alleviation is a wonderful side effect, a silver lining to the Botox procedure, further attesting to the energetic functions of the *Yintang* point, and the physiological workings of acupuncture.

Chapter 15

Luo Points: Special Vessels of Communication Between Channels

Learning Objectives

Luo points are powerful acupuncture points because they can be used in several ways to affect foundational energies. In this chapter the clinician learns how to employ them effectively in clinical practice using both tonification and dispersion techniques and in the Chinese and English methods.

If the body has an inherent wisdom as centuries of Chinese clinical experience suggest that it has, then surely the *Luo* points represent a facet of that wisdom. In classical Chinese acupuncture, *Luo* points are significant vehicles of treatment, although they seem to be less used in modern American acupuncture practice than one would expect given their historical, clinical usefulness. Part of the reason for this fact may be a predilection in American acupuncture colleges to deemphasize the classical energetics of points as discussed in Chapter 8 in favor of a more voluminous litany of point indications. Certainly, these indications are correct, but somehow they have become disassociated from their classical heritage explained through the point classification system. The intent of this chapter is to remind practitioners of the potency of one particular type of Antique point, the *Luo* points, and to demonstrate their value as a treatment option for both tonification and dispersion.

Classical literature reveals that there are three types of *Luos* referred to variously as lesser connecting or contributing channels or collaterals. They are the meridian *Luos* (superficial), the *Blood Luos*, and the minute *Luos*. Each of these *Luos* is a channel or vessel responsible for establishing a network through which *Qi* and *Blood* can be sent to every part of the body.

Minute and *Blood Luos* are very small vessels that arise from the main meridians but are too numerous and too small to be named or conceived of as meridians. They extend to every part of the body and infuse it with the *Qi* and *Blood* of life. Figure 15.1, Meridian, Minute, and *Blood Luos*, depicts a functional image of how these three *Luos* are interconnected and operate in the body.

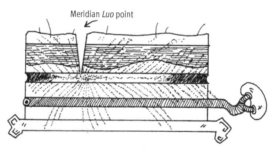

Meridian *Luo* point

Figure 15.1: Meridian, Minute, and Blood Luos

The meridian *Luos* are the *Luo* points of the twelve main meridians. They can be used in two ways. Each way has a different therapeutic aim and each is achieved by a different needle technique. Each *Luo* point activates communication in two directions. One direction relates to the organ–meridian complex that the point is located on and this is known as a longitudinal *Luo*. For instance the Lung *Luo*, LU 7 (*Lieque*), can be used longitudinally to stimulate the Lung organ–meridian. The second pathway connects the particular *Luo* point to the Source point of the coupled organ, and this is known as a transverse *Luo*. In this way, the *Luo* points can be used to internally–externally balance the related organ–meridian complexes. For instance, LU 7 (*Lieque*) can be used transversely to connect to its coupled organ the Large Intestine.

In the case of transverse *Luos*, the *Luo* points of the twelve main meridians connect the *Yin/Yang* pairs and assist in homeostatically regulating the *Yin/Yang* energy between the coupled channels. The *Luo* points do this at the periphery of the superficial skin and muscles before entering the channels. *Luo* points that are used as transverse channels have an oblique trajectory that connects the *Luo* point of a meridian to the Source point of its coupled meridian. In this way, *Luo* points internally-externally connect the coupled organ–meridian complexes so that the *Yin/Yang* organs are connected. When we use the same *Luo* point of the Lung, LU 7 (*Lieque*), as a transverse channel, we communicate between the channels of the husband–wife couple through a special vessel. The *Luo* point allows us to tap into the Source point of the coupled meridian, the Large Intestine.

There are sixteen *Luo* points. Each of the twelve main meridians has a *Luo* point, which is located on the limbs. The *Luo* points of the Conception and Governing Vessel channels are located on the trunk. The Grand *Luo* of the Spleen has an additional *Luo* point, SP 1(*Dabao*), and ST 18 (*Rugen*), another *Luo* on the Stomach meridian, opens to the great channel of the Stomach, another internal pathway between the Stomach and the Heart.

The additional *Luo* points of the Conception and Governing Vessel channels and the Spleen and Stomach channels have other unique functions. At CV 15 (*Jiuwei*), the *Luo* point of the Conception Vessel channel, the *Qi* of all the *Yin* channels converges, and likewise the *Qi* of all of the *Yang* channels concentrates at GV 1 (*Changqiang*), the *Luo* point of the Governing Vessel. All the *Blood* of the body can be activated at SP 21 (*Dabao*), so this point is a handy tonic point particularly in the spring when the dormant energy of winter, the Liver *Qi* and *Blood*, is regenerating and coming to the surface of the body. At ST 18 (*Rugen*) excess Stomach energy may overflow into the upper chest. Sometimes symptoms of heart pain, mistakenly thought of as a heart attack, are maybe indigestion, the overflowing of Stomach energy to the chest through the Stomach *Luo*.

The *Qi* circulates through the superficial skin and muscle layers via the *Luo* channels before entering the primary channels. The connecting channels of the limbs travel toward their respective organs. Those of the Spleen and Stomach spread into the chest, the Conception Vessel disperses into the abdomen, and the Governing Vessel separates into the head and the Bladder channel.

Luo channels are effective in treating chronic disorders of either the organ or its associated meridian. These disorders may be either excess or deficient in nature. The Chinese and the English methods are two primary ways of using *Luo* points for excess and deficient conditions. An analysis of these approaches reveals that the *Luo* points are used quite differently to either tonify or disperse the energy of the organ–meridian complex and yet clinically, each strategy works because they connect *Luo* points to Source points. A comparison and contrast of these methods is summarized in Table 15.1, Interpretations on *Luo* Point Use, for reference.

Table 15.1. Interpretations on *Luo* Point Use

Source	Conditions	Example and Needle Techniques	Explanation	Use
Chinese methods	*Deficiency:* Tonify the Source point of the deficient meridian and disperse the *Luo* point of the coupled meridian *Excess:* For excess in a meridian disperse the *Luo* point of that meridian	*Lung* Qi *deficiency:* Tonify LU 9 (*Taiyuan*), the Source point of the Lung meridian and disperse LI 6 (*Pianli*) the *Luo* point of its couple, the Large Intestine *Lung excess:* Disperse LU7 (*Lieque*), the *Luo* point	Tonification of the Source point strengthens the "source" energy of a meridian. Dispersing the *Luo* point of the coupled channel opens the pathway between the Lung and the Large Intestine such that the husband–wife homeostatic relationship can be achieved Dispersing the *Luo* point of the affected meridian in cases of excess assists in draining excess energy from the meridian	*Transverse* Luo: Angle needle of the *Luo* point toward the Source point and disperse the *Luo* *Longitudinal* Luo: Angle needle along the course of the meridian in either direction with a dispersive technique
English methods	*Deficiency:* In deficiency, Tonify the *Luo* point of the affected meridian and disperse the Source point of the coupled meridian *Excess:* In case of fullness in the meridian, disperse the Source point	*Lung deficiency:* Tonify the *Luo* point LU 7 (*Lieque*) and disperse the Source point of its coupled meridian LI 4 (*Hegu*) *Lung Excess:* Disperse the Source point LU 9 (*Taiyuan*)	Tonifying the *Luo* point is an effective treatment plan whereby to stimulate the organ–meridian complex itself. Dispersing the Source points allows Source energy to be shared with the coupled meridian A treatment strategy to remove excess energy	*Transverse* Luo: Angle needle of the *Luo* point with a dispersive technique toward the Source point to tonify *Longitudinal* Luo: Angle needle along the meridian, opposite the flow of energy to disperse

As with any generalized treatment strategy, be sure that the signs and symptoms fit the clinical picture of the patient and make sense instead of just subscribing to a formula.

CHINESE METHODS

According to the Chinese, the way to use the *Luo* points in cases of deficiency is with their coupled Source point. The rule is as follows: In cases of deficiency, tonify the Source point of the deficient meridian and disperse the *Luo* point of the coupled meridian. An application of this strategy applied to Lung deficiency would be to tonify LU 9 (*Taiyuan*), the Source point of the Lung, the meridian affected by deficiency, and disperse LI 6 (*Pianli*), the *Luo* point of the Large Intestine, the coupled meridian of the Lung.

Most practitioners of Oriental medicine would agree that tonifying the Source point of a deficient meridian to supplement that deficiency makes sense. The added dimension of using *Luo* points may be new and not well understood, but the implication is that by using the *Luo* point to open the channel to the special vessel of communication between channels, homeostatic regulation can be attained between the husband and the wife. This means that the Lung can borrow energy from its *Yang* partner of the same element. If the Large Intestine energy is sufficient or even excessive, it can be related to the Lung, the meridian affected by deficiency. Therefore, disperse LI 6 (*Pianli*), the *Luo* point of the Large Intestine, the coupled meridian of the Lung. A dispersion technique is applied to the point, and the needle is angled along the course of the meridian in either direction. Again, this is a therapeutic approach for dispersing the *Luo* that should make sense to most practitioners. What might be new, but should make sense, is the angle of the needle.

ENGLISH METHODS

Acupuncture, which has its origins in classical Chinese medicine, assumed new nuances as it made its way to England via various countries, translations, and the soil and mind that assimilated it. Like the Chinese, the English use of the *Luo* points has guiding rules for tonifying deficiency and dispersing excess. A look at how they differ is quite useful.

According to the English acupuncture method, the rule is as follows: In deficiency, tonify the *Luo* point of the affected meridian and disperse the Source point of the coupled meridian. Continuing with the case of Lung deficiency, the *Luo* point of the Lung, LU 7 (*Lieque*), would be tonified, and the Source point of its coupled meridian, LI 4 (*Hegu*), would be dispersed.

Analyzing this approach, we see that the meridians are still sharing their energy with each other; the difference lies in what is done to each point. In this system, the *Luo* channel of the deficient meridian is opened and strengthened, and creates a pathway whereby energy from its couple, which is being dispersed, can be brought to it. In this example, the *Luo* point is being used as a transverse vessel, that is, as a channel of communication between the Five Element pairs. To obtain the desired result, needle technique is critical with one point being tonified and another dispersed. In addition, the angle of insertion of the needle is also critical to open up the pathway between the two coupled meridians. In the case of excess in an affected meridian, the rule is, disperse the Source point. Using the example of excess energy in the Lungs, LU 9 (*Taiyuan*), the Source point would be dispersed.

As I have mentioned, the *Luo* points of the twelve main meridians can be used to manipulate either longitudinal or transverse *Luos*. Each has a different therapeutic aim and each is manipulated by a different needle technique. The options are to use the *Luo* channels either longitudinally or transversely. *Luo* points that are used as longitudinal vessels send a stimulus to their corresponding organ by way of the channel. For instance, when LU 7 (*Lieque*), the *Luo* point of the Lungs, is stimulated longitudinally, the needle is inserted obliquely along the course of the Lung meridian in either direction. Which direction to choose would be related to the symptomatology of the meridian. For instance, needle distally if there is a thumb or wrist problem, proximally if the stimulus is to be sent to the Lung organ itself. Treating the point in this way stimulates the Lung organ–meridian complex and this is what using the point as a longitudinal *Luo* means. The sensation along the meridian should be very stimulating.

The Source point is sometimes referred to as the host, and the *Luo* point is termed the guest. Thus, the clinical utility of *Luo* points is either to stimulate the organ–meridian complex proper, or to connect to the Source energy of the coupled meridian. The net effect of such a treatment strategy is an effective clinical approach that can be achieved easily without using too many needles.

We can sometimes observe the diagnostic patterns that the *Luo* points represent. When the *Luo* points are deficient, signs such as flaccidity and indentations can also be noted (Maciocia 1989). We might feel fullness such as rigidity or hardness, see reddish colorations that signify heat, or greenish or whitish colorations indicative of cold retention.

Nguyen Van Nghi, M.D. (verbal, 1986) points out that *Luo* vessels also have discrete channel symptoms that are similar to their organ pathologies and these are very interesting and clinically astute. These symptoms are listed in Table 15.2, Nguyen Van Nghi on *Luo* Point Use. Because they can stimulate the organs and various parts of the body and drain off excesses and supplement deficiency, *Luo* points should be part of every practitioner's repertoire of points.

Table 15.2. Nguyen Van Nghi on *Luo* Point Use

Meridian Symptomatology	Condition	Treatment
Hot palms (heat in hands)	LU fullness	Disperse LU 7 (*Luo*)
Sneezing	LU emptiness	Tonify LU 9 (Source), disperse LI 6 (*Luo*)
Enuresis		
Pain in tooth	LI fullness	Disperse LI 6 (*Luo*)
Coldness in tooth	LI emptiness	Tonify LI 4 (Source), disperse LU 7 (*Luo*)
Craziness, dementia, epilepsy	ST fullness	Disperse ST 40 (*Luo*)
Paralysis	ST emptiness	Tonify ST 42 (Source), disperse SP 4 (*Luo*)
Abdominal colic	SP fullness	Disperse SP 4 (*Luo*)
Swelling of abdomen	SP emptiness	Tonify SP 3 (Source), disperse ST 40 (*Luo*)
Thoracic pain	HT fullness	Disperse HT 5 (*Luo*)
Apnea, can't talk, immobility	HT emptiness	Tonify HT 7 (Source), disperse SI 7 (*Luo*)

(continued)

Meridian Symptomatology	Condition	Treatment
Elbow mobility problems	SI fullness	Disperse SI 7 (*Luo*)
Eczema, furuncles, flaccid paralysis	SI emptiness	Tonify SI 4 (Source), disperse HT 5 (*Luo*)
Nasal obstruction, cephalgia (headache that goes down face) Lumbago	BL fullness	Disperse BL 58 (*Luo*)
	BL emptiness	Tonify BL 64 (Source), disperse KI 4 (*Luo*)
Urinary retention, fecal retention	KI fullness	Disperse KI 4 (*Luo*)
Nosebleed, rhinorrhea	KI emptiness	Tonify KI 3 (Source), disperse BL 58 (*Luo*)
Cardialgia	PC fullness	Disperse PC 6 (*Luo*)
Stiffness in neck	PC emptiness	Tonify PC 7 (Source), disperse TB 5 (*Luo*)
Contraction of elbow	TB fullness	Disperse TB 5 (*Luo*)
Slackness of elbow articulation	TB emptiness	Tonify TB 4 (Source), disperse PC 6 (*Luo*)
Cold feet	GB fullness	Disperse GB 37 (*Luo*)
Laxity at the articulation of the foot	GB emptiness	Tonify GB 40 (Source), disperse LR 5 (*Luo*)
Lengthening of the penis and enlargement of the lips of the vagina	LR fullness	Disperse LR 5 (*Luo*)
	LR emptiness	Tonify LR 3 (Source), disperse GB 37 (*Luo*)
Vaginal or scrotal pruritis		
Stiffness of spine	GV fullness	Disperse GV 1 (*Luo*)
Empty, light-headed, vertigo	GV emptiness	Tonify GV1 (*Luo*)
Painful skin of abdomen	CV fullness	Disperse CV 15 (*Luo*)
Abdominal pruritis, scratching	CV emptiness	Tonify CV 15 (*Luo*)
General pain, a little bit everywhere	Grand *Luo* fullness	Disperse SP 21 (*Luo*)
Superficial on whole body	Grand *Luo* emptiness	Tonify SP 21 (*Luo*)
Laxity of all the joints		

RATIONALE

- For deficiency of a meridian, tonify the Source point of the affected meridian and disperse the *Luo* point of the coupled meridian. Example: If Lung is insufficient, tonify LU 9 (Source point) and disperse LI 6 (*Luo* point) of the coupled meridian. When Large Intestine is deficient, tonify LI 4 (Source point) and disperse LU 7 (*Luo* point) of the Coupled meridian.

- For fullness in a meridian, simply disperse the *Luo* of the meridian.

- Meridians seek equilibrium automatically because of the Chinese clock dynamics, but the use of *Luo* points provides a shortcut to connecting interiorly/exteriorly related organ–meridians.

Summary

The use of *Luo* points is an innate way for the body to regulate its foundational energy and to remove stagnation. Practitioners should be skilled in their use.

Case 7 offers a practical application of the use of a longitudinal *Luo* for excess conditions.

CASE 7: *LUO* POINTS IN EXCESS CONDITIONS

The patient was a forty-two-year-old medical doctor with a diagnosed case of multiple sclerosis. He had many problems that were part of his syndrome. His major complaint centered on extreme, erratic fatigue for the previous seven years. This fatigue was accompanied by several other problems that included the following: 1) leg spasticity and burning pain, 2) lack of bladder control with fluctuations between urgency and a weak stream and/or painful urinary retention, 3) blurry vision and spots before his eyes, 4) loss of balance, and 5) painful constipation and bowel cramps. He had numerous other symptoms, but these were the characteristics of the complaint for which he had sought treatment.

His tongue was red, thin, trembling, and slightly deviated. The sides and tip of the tongue were redder and rough. There were cracks in the Stomach and chest areas. The tongue coat was thick, white, dry, and unrooted. Where there was no coating, the tongue had a glossy or mirror appearance.

His voice was quivery and weak; his lips were pale and sometimes slightly purple. He looked pale, tired, and usually felt hot on palpation. The pulse was slightly fast, deep, thin, and wiry with an irregular missed beat. The Lung, Kidney, and Liver positions were particularly deficient.

Because of the overall deficiency of his condition and the chronic nature of the complaint, I treated this patient for a period of two years, usually on a weekly basis. However, when acute, painful obstructions would develop due to underlying deficiencies, immediate results and relief were required. Under these circumstances, the patient was usually treated several times per week to remedy the condition. Several of these times when the patient complained of certain painful acute conditions, *Luo* points were selected as the points of choice because of their unique attributes.

In one classical usage, *Luo* points were used as channels to drain off or disperse excessive, stuck, or perverse energy. Such excessive energy manifested as prostatitis, a sequela of his urinary disturbance. From time to time his prostate would become enlarged and produce symptoms of referred burning pain to the penis with perineal and suprapubic aching. In addition, he would experience urinary frequency, urgency, and discomfort during urination, difficulty initiating the stream, nighttime urination, and an inability to ejaculate.

When this condition would develop, I tried several different approaches including Chinese herbs, plum blossom needling, and acupuncture, all of which worked. However, the two modalities that had both the most immediate as well as the most long-lasting results included the use of two single points that I used alone or in combination depending upon his situation.

One point was the prostate/uterus point in the ear. On insertion of a needle into this point and a strong dispersion technique, the patient would report that he could immediately feel the burning, achiness, and referred pain diminish. This would occur in less than ten seconds. He would feel very relaxed, even sleepy, and enormously relieved from the pain. To hold the results, I would treat him three days in a row and that time frame appeared successful in setting in motion the reversal of his symptoms.

Another primary treatment point that worked very well was Liver 5 (*Ligou*), the *Luo* point of the Liver channel. To confirm the use of Liver 5 (*Ligou*) as the treatment point I would palpate the point as I do every point that I ever consider needling. Reaction at this point with a strong *Ah Shi* response indicated that the Liver channel was excess or stagnate. Remember that the Liver meridian encircles the external genitalia, hence this is one of the reasons why it was chosen over the *Luo* point of the Bladder or the Kidney. I needled this point in the proximal direction of the meridian, using it as a longitudinal *Luo*, to stimulate the channel, but with a strong dispersion technique to relieve the excess. Many times simply the strong palpation of the point brought about relief, but I always inserted a needle to strengthen the dispersion brought about by the palpation. In this way, the *Luo* point was one of the best points to use for draining the excess from the meridian.

Chapter 16

The Eight Curious Vessels in Oriental Medicine

Learning Objectives ————————————————

In this chapter the pivotal importance of the Curious Vessels is stressed as a way in which to treat the foundational energy of the body, for in essence, the energy they contain is the foundational energy, given at birth, and supplemented through lifestyle factors.

GENERAL FUNCTIONS

The Eight Curious Vessels in Oriental medicine are interesting for the serious student of Eastern medicine who seeks to understand more about bodily energetics and meridian functions. Apart from some esoteric literature, the Eight Curious Vessels, also called the Eight Extra or Extraordinary Meridians, are only superficially understood and used. The purpose of this discussion is to provide the practitioner with a viable, working body of knowledge on this large and important topic.

Nguyen Van Nghi, M.D., the well-known European classical acupuncturist, says that the subject of the Curious Vessels is "not a small idea" (verbal, 1987), referring to the enormity of their physiology. As a result, the discussion in this book is by no means as large as their rich function. Van Nghi suggests, as do I, that these vessels are tools for thinking about bodily energetics. Thus, the Eight Extraordinary Meridians are presented here for the practitioner with this approach in mind. When we use them, we are not treating diseases as much as differentiating syndrome paradigms that match their usage. These are patterns of interaction between the twelve main meridians and other meridian systems. Hence the pathology of a Curious Vessel is characterized by symptoms that encompass several channels.

A search of the available literature reveals that the way the Eight Extraordinary Meridians are used varies somewhat according to the Chinese, European, and Japanese approaches, the cultures that have explored them most intensely. It is my intention to put their crucial functions in the human body into easily understandable terms so beginning students of acupuncture, as well as experienced practitioners, can use these meridians in their practices.

As practitioners know, the Curious Vessels are called by various names: the Eight Extra Meridians, the Eight Extraordinary Meridians, the Eight Secondary Vessels, the Eight Miscellaneous Meridians, and the Eight Psychic Channels. Dr. Van Nghi summarizes their functions in the body and claims that they are not extra, extraordinary, or secondary. Whereas the twelve main meridians may be easier to understand because they have a somewhat Western counterpart, that is, an associated organ, Dr. Van Nghi suggests that the functions of these vessels are indeed curious, and hence he prefers to call them the Eight Curious Vessels. He also maintains that an acupuncture education is seriously deficient and incomplete without understanding them as much as understanding the twelve main meridians

In terms of clinical usage, the Eight Curious Vessels have nine major functions. These functions cover a broad range of disorders that are difficult to treat, as they are often chronic or hard to recognize and hence may require subtle and novel treatment strategies. The Curious Vessels are particularly well suited for these specific disharmonies whose resolution can be more rapid by using them. The nine functions are discussed and summarized in Table 16.1, An Orientation to the Clinical Functions of the Eight Curious Vessels

Table 16.1. An Orientation to the Clinical Functions of the Eight Curious Vessels

Function		Use
Homeostatic	Absorbs excess perverse energy from the twelve main meridians	To treat fever caused by invasion of an exogenous pathogen
Circulatory	Warms and defends the surface by circulating *Wei Qi*	To increase *Yang* in the body
Enriching	Enriches the body with *Qi*, *Blood*, and ancestral *Qi*	To treat deficiencies in those areas
Controlling	Serves as reservoirs and conductors of *Jing*	To treat essence deficiency illness and the developmental life cycle
Nourishing	Harmonizes and nourishes the blood vessels, bone, brain, Gall Bladder, uterus, and bone marrow	To treat diseases of the Liver, Gall Bladder, uterus, brain
Supervisory	Exerts a commanding role over areas of the body, essential substances, and *Zang-fu* organs	To treat zones of the body, essential substances, and *Zang-fu* organs
Balancing	Regulates energy	When the pulses are balanced but the patient still complains of symptoms When the twelve main meridians have failed, and to treat the root causes of a disease
Supplementing	Supplements multiple deficiencies	To treat chronic disease, metabolic and hormonal disorders, psychic strain
Adjusting	Reduces inherited or acquired structural stress	To treat muscle tension, postural or structural stress

1. Homeostatic

The Eight Curious Vessels have a unique capacity as homeostatic vessels. For example, they can absorb excess perverse energy from the twelve main meridians. The perverse energy may be an exogenous, endogenous, or a miscellaneous pathogen or a secondary pathological product. Each Curious Vessel has a Master point which controls it and a Coupled point that activates another Curious Vessel that works well with it. By combining the Master and Coupled points of each set of paired meridians, the Curious Vessels are able to drain or sap these pathogens with remarkable ease. For example, SI 3 (*Houxi*) and BL 6 (*Shenmai*) can be used to treat intermittent fevers caused by an invasion of an exogenous pathogen.

2. Circulatory

Another relationship that the Curious Vessels have with exogenous pathogens is that because the Curious Meridians circulate *Wei Qi*, which warms and defends the surface, they can protect the body from outside invasion. As the "General who Governs the Yang," the Governing Vessel Channel has the particular but not exclusive function of increasing *Wei Qi*.

3. Enriching

The Curious Vessels however are not only adept at annihilating perverse exogenous energy, but they are also able to supply deficiencies and enrich the body with *Qi*, *Blood*, and ancestral *Qi* when the body is weak. As early, structural, formative energies, rich in *Qi* and *Blood*, they are able to do this. They are the internal dynamic of development, the foundational energy of the human body.

4. Controlling

Table 16.2, Origins of the Eight Curious Vessels, summarizes the origins of the Eight Curious Vessels, the conventional thought on their origins. However, in 1985, the World Health Organization agreed that all the Eight Curious Vessels originate in the Kidney but the table is still something to ponder. Thus, the Kidney plays an important role in controlling the development of the body, which it regulates. As a result, the Kidney assumes an important role in controlling the stages of both male and female life cycles discussed at the start of this part of the book under what tonification treatments do.

Table 16.2. Origins of the Eight Curious Vessels

Meridian	Origin
Governing Vessel (GV)	Inside of lower abdomen
Conception Vessel (CV)	Lower abdomen, uterus
Chong (TV)	Uterus, lower abdomen
Dai (DV)	Below the hypochondrium
Yinqiao (YINHV)	Posterior aspect of the navicular bone
Yangqiao (YANGHV)	Lateral side of the heel
Yinwei (YINLV)	Medial side of the leg
Yangwei (YANGLV)	Heel

Many Kidney disorders pertain to the female life cycle of growth, development, and decline and consequently fall within the domain of problems that the Curious Meridians are particularly good at dealing with. Using the Curious Vessels in this manner allows the practitioner to effectively treat the unique physiology and pathology of women. More is said about this in the next chapter, Chapter 17.

The Curious Vessels are rich reservoirs and conductors of *Jing*, the quintessence of energy. As sources of prenatal and postnatal *Qi*, they can supplement the body's energy, making them particularly effective meridians for the treatment of essence deficiency diseases, that is, chronic debilitating illnesses such as early aging, menopause, multiple sclerosis, chronic fatigue, AIDS and any illness not predicated upon the *Qi* cycle for men and women which is a good predictor of declining energy.

5. Nourishing

As conductors of *Jing*, the Eight Curious Vessels nourish the ancestral, extraordinary organs, the blood vessels, bone, brain, Gall Bladder, uterus, and bone marrow. Nourishment of the uterus makes childbearing possible. The Curious Vessels nourish the arteries and circulatory system, the brain, the bones, and marrow, and they harmonize the Liver and Gall Bladder. Diseases of any of these organs, Liver, Gall Bladder, uterus, or brain, or systems such as the hepatobiliary, circulatory, or the skeletal system, can be uniquely treated through the Curious Vessels.

6. Supervisory

The Curious Vessels energetically relate to both the organs and the meridians because they intersect with the twelve main meridians. Because of this connection, they reinforce the points of the twelve regular channels and harmonize the zones between the principal meridians. They thus command or supervise various parts of the body and its functions. For example, the Governing Vessel channel supervises the *Qi* of the primary *Yang* channels and has a strong influence on the Liver, brain, and Kidneys. Table 16.3, The Eight Curious Vessels: Portion of the Body Governed, Physiological Function, and Channel Pathology, illustrates in summary form the physiological functions, physical zones, and meridian symptomatology of the Eight Curious Vessels.

Table 16.3. The Eight Curious Vessels: Portion of the Body Governed, Physiological Function, and Channel Pathology

Meridian	Portion of the Body Governed	Physiological Function	Channel Pathology
Governing Vessel	Neck, shoulders, back, inner canthus	Regulates and stimulates *Yang* energy, increases *Wei Qi*, and circulates the *Yang* of the whole body, for attack by pathogens, particularly wind-cold at the *Taiyang* stage. Supervises the *Qi* of the *Yang* channels. Has strong influence on the Liver. Nourishes the brain, Kidneys, spinal cord. Tends to absorb excess energy from the *Yang* meridians above GV 14 (*Dazhui*) and supply energy to them when they are deficient below GV 14 (*Dazhui*)	Stiffness and pain in spinal column, headache, epilepsy, opisthotonos, diseases of the central nervous system, intermittent fever, *Yang* mental illness (hallucinations), cold, numb extremities, insufficiency of *Wei Qi*

Conception Vessel	Throat, chest, lungs, epigastric region	Concentration of *Yin* energy, controls all the *Yin* meridians. Nourishes the uterus. Absorbs excess energy from *Yin* meridians below CV 8 (*Shenque*) and supplies energy if they are deficient above CV 8 (*Shenque*). For *Yin* and *Blood* problems. Commands diseases related to *Blood* and gynecology	Leukorrhea, irregular menses, hernia, retention of urine, pain in the epigastric region and lower abdomen, infertility in both men and women, nocturnal emission, enuresis, pain in the genitals, rebellious *Qi* in the chest, hormonal problems during menopause and puberty due to stagnation of *Qi* and *Blood*, dysmenorrhea, fibroids, cysts, hot *Blood* problems, chronic itching, pharyngitis, heart disease, stagnation of the whole genital system, genital problems due to stagnation of *Qi* and *Blood*
Chong	Heart, chest, lungs	Arouses Three Leg *Yin* (SP, KI, LR)	Spasm and pain in the abdomen, irregular menstruation, infertility in men and women, asthmatic breathing, removes obstructions and masses, circulates *Blood*, regulates life cycle changes, hormonal sensitivity of uterus, weak digestion from poor constitution with Damp-phlegm accumulation, menstrual problems related to Spleen, stagnation and obstruction

(continued)

Meridian	Portion of the Body Governed	Physiological Function	Channel Pathology
Dai	Retroauricular region, cheek, outer canthus, mastoid region	Promotes pelvic/leg circulation, nourishes hepatobiliary system, supplies deficiencies, influences downward flow of energy. Its disturbances always affect meridians that it encircles at the level of the waist, i.e., SP, ST, KI, Chong, GV, and CV. Its energy depends upon the *Yangming* and GB being sufficient, otherwise the *Dai* is not nourished, leading to pain, paralysis and so on. Controls circulation at the waist and downward	Abdominal pain, weakness and pain of the lumbar area, leukorrhea, hip problems, irregular menses, distention and fullness in the abdomen, prolapse of uterus, muscular atrophy, motor impairment of lower extremities, migraines
Yinqiao	Lower abdomen, lumbar, and hip area, pubis	Brings fluid and *Jing* to the eyes, secondary vessel of the Kidney	Hypersomnia, *Yin* deficiency especially at night, spasm of lower limbs, inversion of foot, epilepsy, lethargy, pain in the lower abdomen, pain in the lumbar region and hip referring to the pubis, problems of eyes, genitals, bone marrow, genital stagnation; used mainly for women
Yangqiao	Inner canthus, back, lumbar region, lower limbs	Secondary vessel to the Bladder, absorbs excess energy of head (brain, eyes)	Epilepsy, insomnia, redness and pain of inner canthus, pain in back, lumbar region, eversion of foot, spasms of lower limbs
Yinwei	Interior syndromes	Preserver of the *Yin*; principal vessel of the Kidney; binds the *Yin*	Cardialgia, chest pain, all *Yin* deficiency especially of the Heart
Yangwei	Exterior syndromes	Preserver of the *Yang*; binds all *Yang* meridians	Chills and fever, imbalance in defensive energy

7. Balancing

Because of the energetic relationships between the organs and all of the meridians, the use of the Eight Curious Vessels facilitates treatment of the root cause of a disease regardless of its etiology. Therefore the Eight Curious Vessels can be used when the twelve main meridians have failed. This is an important feature to keep in mind for sometimes practitioners cannot successfully treat disorders only using the twelve main meridians.

As the precursors to the twelve main meridians, the Curious Vessels regulate their *Qi* and *Blood*. Therefore, the Eight Curious Vessels can be used when the pulses are balanced but the patient still complains of symptoms. In this case, the patient's signs and symptoms must correspond to Eight Curious Vessel pathology.

8. Supplementing

When a multiplicity of deficiencies points in the same direction, for example, generalized *Yin* deficiency, *Yang* deficiency, or specific organ deficiency such as Kidney *Qi* deficiency, or a combination of *Qi* deficiencies such as Lung *Qi*, Kidney *Qi*, Spleen *Qi* and so on, the Eight Curious Vessels may be employed. Other examples include chronic disease, depleted energy, metabolic and hormonal disorders, mental/psychological strain, or when too many needles would weaken the patient.

9. Adjusting

For palpable or spontaneous muscle tension and postural or structural stress that is either inherited or acquired, the Eight Curious Meridians are particularly well-suited because they are the outlines of the earliest formative energies created just after conception. They are the first primordial meridians, the infrastructure of who we are and what we may become. Their existence predates the *Zang-fu*, the tendinomuscular meridians, the *Luo*, and the divergent meridians. They are the fundamental source of our bodily armor as well as the genetic basis of who we are and how we may develop. They were formed immediately after the fertilization of the egg, with the first cell division creating the

Conception Vessel and Governing Vessel channels, and thereafter with each progressive cell division, that made up the blastomere. As such, they are particularly beneficial in the treatment of both inherited as well as acquired musculoskeletal disorders.

Table 16.4, Additional Meanings of the Names of the Curious Vessels, offers a unique view on how to use these vessels by looking at an interpretation of their Chinese characters. Keep in mind that Chinese characters are not static but energetic symbols and have many meanings. This vision offered by Kiiko Matsumoto (1986, p.3) provides valuable insight into their clinical use. Finally, Table 16.5, A Summary of the Eight Curious Vessels: Significant Points and Treatment Approaches, gives a summary of the Eight Curious Vessels, their significant points, and treatment approaches.

Table 16.4. Additional Meanings of the Names of the Curious Vessels

Meridian	Name
Governing Vessel	General who governs *Yang*. The sea of various *Yang Chings*
Conception Vessel	Pregnancy, obligation. To accept or hold something in front of the abdomen. The sea of *Yin* meridians
Chong	Street. Used to express the idea of passing or transformation, alchemical transformation, two entities clashing together to produce something different. Assault, what goes up
Dai	Belt. Acts as support, bundles all the meridians together
Wei	Rope tied around something. It pulls down and secures. Controls downward movement. Preserver of *Yin* or *Yang*, particularly *Yin* and *Yang* defensive energy

Table 16.5. A Summary of the Eight Curious Vessels:
Significant Points and Treatment Approaches

Meridian	Meaning of Name	Master Points	Coupled Points	*Xi* (Cleft)/ *Luo* Points*	Coalescent Points
Du Mai (GV)	Governor vessel. Governs all *Yang* channels	SI 3 (*Houxi*)	BL 62 (*Shenmai*)	GV 1* (*Changxiang*)	X
Ren Mai (CV)	Conception Vessel. Responsible to all *Yin* channels and nourishes the fetus	LU 7 (*Lieque*)	KI 6 (*Zhaohai*)	CV 15* (*Jiuwei*)	X

Chong Mai (TV)	Sea of *Blood*, Sea of Arteries and Meridians, Thoroughfare Vessel, Penetrating Vessel. Vital channel communicating with all the channels; regulates the *Qi* and *Blood* of the twelve regular meridians	SP 4 (*Gongsun*)	PC 6 (*Neiguan*)	X	CV 1 (*Huiyin*) KI 11–21 (see the Point Index for names)
Dai Mai (DV)	Belt Vessel, Girdle Channel. Binds all the channels	GB 41 (*Zulinqi*)	TB 5 (*Waiguan*)	X	GB 26 (*Daimai*), GB 27 (*Wushu*), GB 28 (*Weidao*)
Yinqiao Mai (YINHV)	*Yin* Heel Vessel, Heel agility, Accelerator of the *Yin*	KI 6 (*Shaohai*)	LU 7 (*Lieque*)	KI 8 (*Jiaoxin*)	KI 6 (*Shaohai*), KI 8 (*Jiaoxin*)
Yangqiao Mai (YANGHV)	*Yang* Heel Vessel, Accelerator of the *Yang*	BL 62 (*Shenmai*)	SI 3 (*Houxi*)	BL 59 (*Fuyang*)	BL 1 (*Jingmeng*) BL 59 (*Fuyang*), BL 61 (*Pucan*), BL 62 (*Shenmai*) GB 20 (*Fengchi*), GB 29 (*Juliao*), SI 10 (*Noash*) ST 4 (*Dicang*), ST 3 (*Juliao*), ST 1 (*Chengqi*), LI 15 (*Jianyu*), LI 16 (*Jugu*)
Yinwei Mai (YINLV)	*Yin* Link Vessel. Connects with all *Yin* channels	PC 6 (*Neiguan*)	SP 4 (*Gongsun*)	KI 9 (*Zubin*)	KI 9 (*Zubin*), SP 13 (*Fushe*), SP 15 (*Daheng*), SP 16 (*Fuai*), LR 14 (*Qimen*), CV 22 (*Tiantu*), CV 23 (*Lianquan*)
Yangwei Mai (YANGLV)	*Yang* Link Vessel. Connects with all *Yang* channels	TB 5 (*Waiguan*)	GB 41 (*Zulinqi*)	GB 35 (*Yangqiao*)	BL 63 (*Jinmen*), GB 35 (*Yangqiao*), GB 13–21 (see the Point Index for names), GV 15 (*Yamen*), GV 16 (*Fengfu*), ST 8 (*Touwei*), SI 10 (*Noashu*), TB 15 (*Tianliao*)

Summary

The Eight Curious Vessels play many important roles in the human body. When the information herein and these charts are understood, the practitioner will find they are using the Curious Vessels frequently in the treatment of foundational energies.

APPLICATIONS OF THE EIGHT CURIOUS VESSELS: *JING* TREATMENTS

As noted, one important use of the Eight Curious Vessels is when a number of deficiencies point in the same direction. As practitioners of Chinese medicine know, deficiency is a common clinical condition. New types of illness characterized as essence deficiency diseases are becoming more common from environmental contamination, poor food quality, cultural stress, and prescription drugs. When a patient presents with multiple deficiencies, it is often difficult to decide where to begin to treat. Also, these people are weak and rarely tolerate many needles. Multiple deficiencies often present as chronic fatigue, fibromyalgia, AIDS, and multiple sclerosis, amongst others. In these cases the Chinese *Jing* treatment can be beneficial.

The Chinese *Jing* treatment consists of needling the Eight Confluent points, that is, the Master points of the Eight Curious Vessels and CV 6 (*Qihai*). Needles are inserted from top to bottom beginning with the Master point of one meridian and its corresponding coupled meridian. I prefer to open the *Dai* meridian first as it is the only horizontal meridian and as such functionally binds all the twelve main meridians and the remaining Curious Vessels together. If the *Dai* meridian is obstructed, it can bind the other meridians in a dysfunctional manner and hence it is useful to open it at the start of treatment. *Dai* meridian obstructions can develop from poor posture, excess weight, organ prolapses, tight clothing, pregnancy, and wearing high heels. Opening the *Dai* channel is accomplished by needling TB 5 (*Waiguan*), usually on the right side, and then complementing this point by needling its Coupled point, GB 41 (*Zulinqi*), on the left. This strategy corresponds to the strategy for unilateral needling discussed throughout this book and found in Table 16.6, Unilateral Needling, derived from historical pulse systems found in the classics, as set out in Table 16.7.

Table 16.6. Unilateral Needling
General rule of thumb – Which side of the body to needle in unilateral needling is based upon pulse assignments

Right	Left
LU	HT
LI	SI
SP	BL
ST	PC
TB	LR
None	GB
KI	KI

Table 16.7. A Historical Comparison of Various Pulse Diagnosis Systems

Pulse Systems	Position	Right Hand			Left Hand		
		Distal	*Middle*	*Proximal*	*Distal*	*Middle*	*Proximal*
Yellow Emperor's Classic (*Neijing*) ca. 200 B.C.	Superficial Deep	Chest LU	SP ST	Abdomen KI	Sternum HT	Diaphragm LR	Abdomen KI
Five Element Classic (*Nanjing*) ca. 200 B.C.	Superficial Deep	LI LU	ST SP	TB PC	SI HT	GB LR	BL KI
Wang Shu-he: Pulse Classic ca. 280 B.C.	Superficial Deep	LI LU	ST SP	TB MM*	SI HT	GB LR	BL KI
Li Shi-zhen: Pulse Diagnosis A.D. 1564	Middle	LU	SP	MM* and LI, TB	HT	LR	MM*, SI, BL
Zhang Jie-bing: Complete Book A.D. 1624	Superficial Deep	Sternum LU	ST SP	TB, MM*, SI, KI	PC HT	GB LR	BL, LI KI
Eight Principle Pulse system	Superficial Deep	LU -	ST SP	- KI *Yang*	HT -	GB LR	- KI *Yin*
Contemporary China based on the classics	Superficial Deep	LI, chest LU	ST SP	LI, TB, MM*	PC HT	GB LR	SI, BL KI

*MM: *Mingmen* (Gate of Life) = Kidney *Yin* and *Yang* immutably bound together
Source: International Training Center of the Academy of Traditional Chinese Medicine, Beijing, 1988, 1989

Next, I highly recommend needling PC 6 (*Neiguan*) on the left as a primary point to move any stagnation. I believe that stagnation should be relieved before deficiencies are tonified so that any zonal blockages are not correspondingly or inadvertently tonified, that is, strengthened or exacerbated. SP 4 (*Gongsun*), the Coupled point to PC6 (*Neiguan*), is subsequently needled on the right side. PC 6 (*Neiguan*) is the point to move stagnation anywhere in the body, particularly in the Upper *Jiao*.

LU 7 (*Lieque*) on the right and KI 6 (*Zhaohai*) on the left are then needled, followed by SI 3 (*Houxi*) on the left and BL 62 (*Shenmai*) on the right. Finally, CV 6 (*Qihai*) is inserted.

Some practitioners have reported that the order of needle insertion is not critical to the effectiveness of treatment, but the point is to have a reason for what you do. Just as I have done, the practitioner is encouraged to monitor and evaluate clinical results for the benefit of the patient with whichever way you execute treatment. The protocol presented here is my preferred treatment strategy.

Excellent technique when inserting and manipulating the needle is imperative to avoid pain at these points as well as to achieve the desired result. Needles should be retained from ten to thirty minutes depending on the patient's condition. Start with shorter time periods to assess how the patient reacts and then as the patient gets stronger, the needles can be retained for a longer time. The weaker the patient, the shorter the retention time.

This treatment works on a very deep energetic level. As a result, when being needled, it is not uncommon for the patient to experience a state of relaxation instead of being superficially energized. Patients may desire to rest further after the treatment and they should be encouraged to wait until they feel ready before leaving the office. In addition, they should be advised not to expend energy unnecessarily so that the vital *Qi* contacted during the treatment is allowed to consolidate at a deeper level.

Sometimes practitioners are concerned that they should not use the Eight Curious Vessels at all or infrequently. However, a review of their multiple and important functions, as well as clinical experience, does not discourage and in fact supports their careful use. Table 16.8, Eight Confluent Point Protocol, summarizes the Eight Confluent point protocol in terms of point location, angle and depth of insertion, needling, and palpation technique.

Table 16.8. Eight Confluent Point Protocol

Point Order	Eight Curious Vessel Master Point	Coupled Point	Side of Body to Palpate/Needle	Palpation Method	Sensation	Point Location	Needle Technique (Japanese Needles Best #1 30mm)
TB 5 (Waiguan)	Yangwei Mai	GB 41 (Zulinqi)	Right side	Deep palpation to PC 6 (Neiguan) perpendicular pressure. Relatively speaking palpation on this side will be more shallow because Yang side is more muscular and Yin more mushy	Not as strong as subsequent points but when relevant, patient perceives sensation at the point	Standard TB 5 location	Perpendicular superficial insertion .3 in. No or small manipulation depending upon patient's constitution
GB 41 (Zulinqi)	Dai Mai	TB 5 (Waiguan)	Left side	Vigorous rubbing	Point is shallow and extremely painful in general	Two locations: standard GB 41 (Zulinqi) location and Japanese location in the depression anterior to the cuboid bone	For either location, obliquely .3 in. in the direction of the meridian (towards the toe)
PC 6 (Neiguan)	Yinwei Mai	SP 4 (Gongsun)	Left side	Deep perpendicular palpation to TB 5 (Waiguan)	Very tender when pathological	Standard PC 6 (Neiguan) location	Superficial insertion .3 in. No or light manipulation depending upon patient's constitution
SP 4 (Gongsun)	Chong Mai	PC 6 (Neiguan)	Right side	Solid rub against the bone	Extremely painful in most cases	Standard SP 4 (Gongsun) location	Perpendicular or oblique insertion .3 in. If oblique, needle in direction of meridian (towards the heel)
LU 7 (Lieque)	Ren Mai	KI 6 (Zhaohai)	Right side	Push against bone	Not much comes up on palpation because of the size of the point but it can. Other signs and symptoms will support the use of the point	Standard LU 7 (Lieque) location	Obliquely .3 in. in direction of the meridian (towards the thumb). Sometimes I go up the arm for dispersion

KI 6 (*Zhaohai*)	*Yinqiao Mai*	Both sides	With thumb push into the point	Characteristically tender, usually more on one side than other, choose most tender	One of the alternate Chinese locations defined as 1 *cun* below medial malleolus, but slightly superior to the junction of the red and the white skin in a depression generally marked with a (X) fold in the skin	Posteriorly horizontally .1–2 in. in direction of meridian (towards the heel)
SI 3 (*Houxi*)	*Du Mai*	Left side	Obliquely upward against the bone	In terms of frequency does not come up that often, except when indicated and then there is some sensation that the patient reports	Standard SI 3 (*Houxi*) location	Perpendicular or obliquely upward (towards the fingers) .2 in.–3 in.
BL 62 (*Shenmai*)	*Yangqiao Mai*	Right side	This is a shallow point; firmly rub it	Generally very sore	Japanese BL 62 location which is closer to the Chinese BL 61 location	Obliquely .2 in.–3 in. in the direction of the meridian (towards the toes)
CV 6 (*Qihai*)	X	Center	In pathology, either a sensation of mushiness indicative of deficiency or hardness which is excess due to underlying deficiency. Resilient and good tone in health	Dislike if in pathology, sometimes invasive and guarded	On the midline of the abdomen 1.5 *cun* below the center of the umbilicus	Perpendicularly 1 in.–1.5 in. Summon *Qi* to the area and tonify

Chapter 17

The Clinical Significance of the Confluent Points and Their Applications in Gynecology

Learning Objectives

This chapter is devoted to the clinical significance of the Confluent points so that the practitioner can understand the unique energetics of each one. Because many of these functions have a positive effect on women's health, the application of these points to gynecological issues is stressed.

THE CONFLUENT POINTS
TB 5 (*Waiguan*)

The *Luo* point of the Triple Burner meridian is TB 5 (*Waiguan*). It maintains the critical function of connecting all three *Jiaos*, or burning spaces, where the essential substances of *Qi*, *Blood*, *Jing*, and *Body* fluids (*Jin-ye*) are both created and harmoniously distributed to every part of the body for use or storage. Tenderness elicited at this point by palpation can indicate problems with digestion and elimination. These problems can be stagnation from digestive pathology or the presence of the pathological by-products of Phlegm, Damp, and stagnant *Blood* in one or more of the *Jiaos*. Gynecological manifestations of these pathological by-products include leukorrhea, cysts, abdominal accumulations, and tumors of a benign or malignant nature.

Wei means "connection." TB 5 (Waiguan) translated as the Outer Gate, that is, as the Master of the Yangwei Mai (Yang defensive system), mobilizes the Yang defensive energies of the body. It connects all the Yang channels that assist in protecting the organism. As Master point of the Yangwei channel, TB 5 (Waiguan) commands the outside of the body. Tenderness at this point may indicate a weakness in the Yang organ–meridian systems or weakness in the True Qi of the body that protects the person from outside evils. Thus, exterior syndromes are governed by TB 5 (Waiguan). Palpable tenderness at this site may also indicate the tendency to be easily invaded by exogenous pathogens, which can further weaken the body's True Qi because of the constant battle between the antipathogenic factor and the evil Qi. It is a useful point for gynecological problems caused by exogenous invasion such as dysmenorrhea due to external cold.

GB 41 (Zulinqi)

GB 41 (Zulinqi) is a primary point for women's health problems because of its intimate relationship to the Liver and the Dai channel. The Gall Bladder, as the Yang functional counterpart of the Liver, can be viewed as an accurate index of Liver Yang rising. In terms of gynecological function, this point is excruciatingly tender on palpation when the patient has Liver Yang rising, because of Liver Yin or Liver Blood deficiency, or if the patient has Liver Qi and/or Liver Blood stagnation. When GB 41 (Zulinqi) is tender, women are prone to scanty menses, cramps, breast tenderness, fibrocystic breasts, irritability, and migraine headache. There may be premenstrual symptoms such as fatigue with the period, cravings for salt or other stimulants like chocolate, coffee, or spicy food that temporarily decongest Liver Qi. Also, there can be mild back pain, constipation, and weakened vision.

GB 41 (Zulinqi) may also be sensitive if Liver Qi is invading earth. As a result of wood overacting on earth, when wood is excessive, the Spleen Qi usually becomes deficient. Damp accumulates and Blood is not produced. Also, the Stomach can become hot as a result of this overacting cycle. Stomach Yin is consumed and Damp and Phlegm develop. GB 41 (Zulinqi) is a Yang point that can reflect the condition of the Yin, particularly the Yin deficiencies of the Liver, Kidney, and Stomach.

As the Horary point and wood point of the Gall Bladder meridian, GB 41 (*Zulinqi*) promotes the free flow of Liver *Qi*. It is beneficial in resolving Dampness in the genital region such as leukorrhea, and in clearing Phlegm-heat and stagnant *Blood* that can cause symptoms of abdominal stagnation such as endometriosis and dysmenorrhea.

GB 41 (*Zulinqi*) is the Master point of the *Dai* channel, the one meridian that encircles, bundles, and ties all the meridians together as the body's only horizontal support system. Its disturbances are harmful to the meridians it surrounds at the level of the waist which are the Gall Bladder, Spleen, Stomach, Kidney, *Chong* channel, Conception Vessel, and Governing Vessel channels. Consequently, it regulates the *Jiaos* above and below its pathway, influences leg and pelvic circulation, and contributes to the nourishment of the hepatobiliary system.

The health of the *Dai* channel depends on the ability of the Gall Bladder and *Yangming* energy (Stomach/Large Intestine layer) to create ample *Qi* and *Blood*. Gynecologically, the *Dai* channel is implicated in irregular menses, leukorrhea, scanty menses, painful periods, and edema of the Lower *Jiao*.

Clinically, TE 5 (*Waiguan*) and GB 41 (*Zulinqi*) work together synergistically. As depicted in Figure 17.1, Image of the Functional Relationship between TB 5 (*Waiguan*) and GB 41 (*Zulinqi*), we can see the relationship between these two meridians, *Yangwei* and *Dai*. It can be compared to a spiral that encompasses all three *Jiaos* longitudinally and latitudinally.

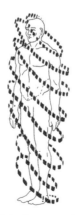

Figure 17.1: Image of the Functional Relationship between
*TB 5 (*Waiguan*) and GB 41 (*Zulinqi*)*

PC 6 (*Neiguan*)

PC 6 has strong connections to gynecological health. These energetics are described herein.

- *Neiguan* as a *Luo* (Connecting) point.

- According to Chinese medicine, *Luo* points can be used as openings either to the transverse or to the longitudinal vessels. As a transverse *Luo*, a stimulus can be sent to the coupled organ–meridian complex, in this case, the *San Jiao*, the Triple Burner. Through the longitudinal *Luo*, *Neiguan* stimulates its own organ–meridian complex through the internal pathway of the channel.

- *Neiguan* as the Master Point of the *Yinwei* channel.

- As the master point of all the *Yin* organ–meridian complexes, the Lung, Heart, Pericardium, Liver, Spleen, and Kidney, *Neiguan* links them together.

- In the Six Division framework, *Neiguan* is bound to the Liver at the *Jueyin* level.

- *Neiguan* coupled with the *San Jiao* in the Five Elements.

- The use of *Neiguan* to assess the immune function derives from the fact of its connection to the Triple Burner, which thereby connects it to the entire metabolism of the body.

- Pericardium–Uterus–Kidney Relationship.

- There is a connection from the Pericardium to the Kidney and from the Kidney to the uterus. This gives *Neiguan* considerable influence in gynecological issues. This is depicted in Figure 17.2, Pericardium, Uterus, and Kidney Relationship.

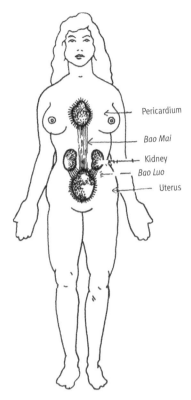

Figure 17.2: Pericardium, Uterus, and Kidney Relationship

- Coupled with the *Chong* channel and its Confluent Point in the Eight Extra Vessel System.

- The *Chong* channel and its Master point, SP 4 (*Gongsun*) are coupled in the Eight Extra Vessel system with the *Yinwei* channel governed by PC 6 (*Neiguan*).

- All the Eight Curious Vessels meet at PC 6 (*Neiguan*).

- Because all of the Eight Extra Meridians meet at *Neiguan*, this fact alone makes the point extremely important for the immune system and gynecological health by regulating *Yin, Yang, Qi, Blood* and *Jing*.

SP 4 (*Gongsun*)

Spleen 4 (*Gongsun*) is the *Luo* point of the Spleen organ–meridian complex. In this capacity, SP 4 (*Gongsun*) is useful in coordinating the functional relationship between the Spleen and the Stomach. It tonifies, pacifies, and regulates Spleen and Stomach disharmony, removes turbidity and obstruction, and circulates *Qi* and *Blood*. SP 4 (*Gongsun*) is useful in clearing obstructions of Dampness from the Spleen, which can lead to cysts or leukorrhea. Additionally, it can quell fire in the Stomach that consumes *Yin* and causes scanty menses, amenorrhea, and infertility.

Perhaps the most consistently painful point in the body, SP 4 (*Gongsun*), is exquisitely tender in patients with Spleen *Qi* deficiency, Damp accumulation, and *Blood* deficiency patterns. These symptoms are characteristic of people who overwork, eat irregularly, worry excessively, or have poor nutritional patterns. Obviously, Spleen *Qi* is essential for the sound energy of the entire body and gynecological health in particular because of its role in *Blood* production and regulation. As a reactive point, SP 4 (*Gongsun*) can indicate *Blood* deficiency manifesting as scanty menses or as premenstrual syndrome (PMS), symptoms of headache, amenorrhea, backache, or dysmenorrhea from Liver *Qi* stagnation arising out of Liver *Blood* deficiency.

Spleen 4 (*Gongsun*) is the Master point of the *Chong* meridian and the Coupled point of the *Yinwei* channel. It is coupled energetically to PC 6 (*Neiguan*). The *Chong* meridian, translated variously as the "thoroughfare vessel," "the vital channel," "the sea of arteries and meridians," but more commonly known as the Sea of Blood, summarizes the role of the *Chong* as a reservoir of *Blood* created by the joint efforts of the Spleen and Kidney. The *Chong*, like the Spleen and Kidney, flows upward, bringing with it the products of *Qi*, *Blood*, and *Jin-ye* (Body fluid). It regulates the *Qi* and *Blood* of the twelve regular channels and arouses the Three Leg *Yin*. PC 6 (*Neiguan*) and SP 4 (*Gongsun*) work closely and homeostatically together to produce and distribute the basic body substances to every part of the body.

LU 7 (*Lieque*)

LU 7 (*Lieque*), the *Luo* connecting point of the Lung meridian, has the ability to tonify the *Qi* of the Lungs and therefore of the whole body because the Lungs are the Master of the *Qi*. As a *Luo* point, it sustains the energy of the whole body and is classically viewed as a general tonic point. It is also effective in dissipating water from the body. It stimulates its coupled organ, the Large Intestine, to do its job of being the Great Eliminator. It removes the dregs that may deteriorate into pathological stagnation in the body. By virtue of its *Luo* point function and internal pathway, the Lung meridian opens up the chest and sends its *Qi* downward to be grasped by the Kidney. It is useful for rebellious *Qi* in the chest and is actually one of the best points for rebellious *Qi*. Dispersion of LU 7 (*Lieque*) as a *Luo* point will break up Dampness or Phlegm in the Lungs.

Lung 7 (*Lieque*) is the Master of the Conception Vessel (*Ren*) channel. *Ren* means responsibility and the CV channel is responsible to all the *Yin* channels. It is an extremely efficient point for opening the CV channel so its energy can flow upward. LU 7 (*Lieque*) affects all the points on the CV channel including the *Mu* points of the Pericardium, Heart, Stomach, Triple Burner, Kidney, Small Intestine, Bladder, and other points on the CV channel that have important energetics. It passes through the uterus and nourishes the fetus. Gynecological problems from stagnant *Qi* or *Blood* such as fibroids, painful periods, and cysts are well treated with LU 7 (*Lieque*). The CV channel is effective in absorbing excess energy from the *Yin* meridians below CV 8 (*Shenque*) and it can supply energy to the *Yin* meridians if they are deficient above CV 8 (*Shenque*).

KI 6 (*Zhaohai*)

KI 6 (*Zhaohai*) is one of the most important points of the body, in some Japanese schools of thought perhaps the most important point. Its major function is to add *Yin* to the body and it is generally considered the best point with which to nourish *Yin*. It is extremely tender in patients with *Yin* deficiency. As a *Yin* point, it is useful for cooling the *Blood* and for promoting uterine and hormonal function. KI 6 (*Zhaohai*) benefits the Kidney and strengthens vital essence.

One of the most common etiologies of *Jing* and *Yin* deficiency is stress. KI 6 (*Zhaohai*) is considered to be the point that best indicates and treats Kidney *Yin* deficiency. It is called the adrenal reflex point and denotes the effects of shock, trauma, chronic diseases, and lifestyle factors that have consumed *Yin*.

As the Master of the *Yinqiao* channel, KI 6 (*Zhaohai*) controls the distribution of *Yin* energy to the upper part of the body, including the eyes. The *Yinqiao* channel ends at BL 1 (*Jingming*). KI 6 (*Zhaohai*) is useful for heat arising out of *Yin* deficiency and fatigue. Gynecologically, it can be used to treat early period, menopause, premature graying, hot flashes, personality disturbances, chronic illness, and dry eyes, all signs of Kidney *Yin* and essence deficiency.

Lung 7 (*Lieque*) is coupled with Kidney 6 (*Zhaohai*). The Lungs send their energy down and the Kidney grasps that *Qi* and propels it upward as depicted in Figure 17.3, Lung and Kidney Relationship. The image of the two channels together is similar to a wheel that puts stagnation in motion.

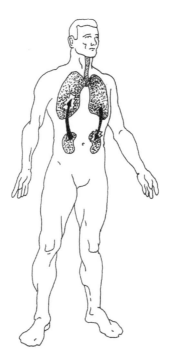

Figure 17.3: Lung and Kidney Relationship

SI 3 (*Houxi*)

SI 3 (*Houxi*) is the *Shu* (stream) point, the wood point, and the tonification point of the Small Intestine meridian. It is clinically effective for joint, bone and neck, and muscle and tendon problems. These symptoms frequently accompany essence deficiency diseases like menopause and infertility.

In Japanese acupuncture, SI 3 (*Houxi*) is considered a point that indicates the health of the pituitary gland (verbal, Matsumoto 1988). Though it is somewhat awkward to palpate, a positive response can be elicited at the point. SI 3 (*Houxi*) is an effective point for gynecological problems connected to the pituitary gland, the master gland of the body, which is responsible for hormonal regulation. Women with a tender SI 3 (*Houxi*) often have gynecological problems diagnosed as Kidney *Yang* deficiency or stagnant *Blood* arising from the use of birth control pills, which alter the hormonal environment of the user and cause Liver *Qi* and *Blood* stagnation (Flaws 1990).

Small Intestine 3 (*Houxi*) is the Master point of the Governing Vessel channel. As the Master point that governs all the *Yang* channels, it aids in regulating the *Yang* energy that arises upward via the Governing Vessel channel. Thus, it affects the flow of energy from the Kidney through the spine, neck, head, and face. It increases the Yang of the whole body.

BL 62 (*Shenmai*)

BL 62 (*Shenmai*) is the Master point of the *Yangqiao* channel. It is responsible for absorbing excess *Yang* energy in the upper part of the body all the way to the eyes, thus holding it down. Excess energy in the upper part of the body in the form of headache, personality disturbances, insomnia, and hot flashes that may accompany menopause can be treated with BL 62 (*Shenmai*). Governing Vessel energy manipulated by using SI 3 (*Houxi*) lifts energy from the lower part of the body. This is the image of how these two points work together.

Although BL 62 (*Shenmai*) is coupled with SI 3 (*Houxi*), it can be used gynecologically with KI 6 (*Zhaohai*). This is an effective combination for the hot flashes associated with menopause, particularly if the patient also has signs and symptoms of underlying Kidney *Yin* deficiency. The combination of these points regulates the *Yin* and *Yang* energy of the heel vessel that travels to the head. These points together absorb excess energy in that area. The treatment consists of tonifying KI 6 (*Zhaohai*), and dispersing BL 62 (*Shenmai*).

Summary

We see that the Confluent points possess energetics that are widely applicable to the treatment of gynecological problems as well as other conditions. They can be needled singularly, in combination with their coupled Confluent point, or used as the skeletal basis of treatment. The palpation and needling of the Eight Confluent points can be found in Table 16.8, on the Eight Confluent Point Protocol, in Chapter 16. Case 8 illustrates the use of Confluent points in the treatment of menopause.

CASE 8: THE TREATMENT OF MENOPAUSE WITH THE EIGHT CURIOUS VESSELS

The patient was a forty-seven-year-old-female whose major complaint was of menopausal symptoms that had begun two weeks previously. The signs and symptoms included hot flashes, dull hot abdominal pain, hip pain, feelings of delusion and disorientation, night sweats, extreme thirst, occipital headaches, itchy skin, depression and sadness, fatigue, worry, heavy limbs, poor sleep, facial breakouts, lots of gas, neck and back pain, canker sores, dream-disturbed sleep, and constipation. She had been taking estrogen therapy for those two weeks, but had decided to discontinue it because of a history of fibrocystic tumors in both herself and her family.

The tongue was pale, swollen, and short with a red tip and sides, a thick, yellow, greasy coat, and a central crack. She had thick, coarse, gray hair. Her lips were purple, the face dry and wrinkled. Her body was short and stocky and she wore tight jewelry and tight clothing. The pulse was weak, thready, and rapid on the left and slippery on the right.

From age and a lifestyle that included a lot of stress, and from poor nutrition and lots of alcohol consumption, the *Qi* of the Kidney was weak. The patient manifested signs and symptoms of Kidney *Qi* deficiency, that is both *Yin* and *Yang* deficiency, and that produced symptoms of heat and cold with *Blood* deficiency. This further led to symptoms of Heart *Blood* deficiency and Spleen *Qi* deficiency.

The diagnosis was depletion of Kidney essence, Liver *Blood* and *Yin* deficiency, Liver *Qi* stagnation, Heart *Blood* deficiency, and Spleen *Qi* deficiency. The etiology and pathogenesis of her case was from the natural decline of Kidney *Qi* exacerbated by stress, diet, lifestyle factors, alcohol, and her underlying constitution. The treatment plan was to tonify the Kidney essence and to tonify the *Qi* and the *Blood*.

To get a sense of the whole person, as well as the complexity of the case, I have provided the answers to the Ten Questions and observations that represent pathological data:

- depression, agitated, weepy, overreacts, "craziness," "spaciness," disorientation

- facial breakouts

- shoulders frequently hurt, pain at the vertex, neck tension, headaches at *Taiyang*

- on synthroid for multiple goiters from forty years of age

- two fibrocystic tumors in left breast

- history of erratic periods, once spotted for two months

- darkness under the eyes

- pain in the inguinal region

- lower lumbar/sacral pain at the iliac crest, sciatic pain

- craves salads, vegetables, eats lot of frozen yogurt, periodically eats spoiled food

- feeling of organs sinking

Acupuncture was administered for a period of ten weeks, two times a week. The treatment improved the hip pain, eliminated the headaches and the abdominal pain, cooled the skin, calmed the spirit, reduced the hot flashes and the insomnia, and improved mood. There had been an adverse reaction to herbs in the past with another practitioner and the patient was hesitant to try herbs again.

However, herbs were introduced into therapy in the third week and they further diminished the hot flashes. At this point a correlation could always be made between the hot flashes and stress.

The patient was very compliant in receiving treatments on a regular basis and only took the herbs because of her trust in the practitioner. She was reluctant to change her lifestyle habits of late nights, drinking alcohol, tight clothing, and did not take measures to reduce stress. As of the last follow-up, ten months after treatment stopped, the patient relied only upon one herbal tablet per day to control the hot flashes. Her nipples changed from post pregnancy brown to the color of a young girl's! Mental symptoms subsided after six treatments. Fourteen treatments improved tongue color to a light red, reduced its flabbiness, cleared the thick, yellow greasy coat to thin white, and eliminated all symptoms, reducing the hot flashes from five times an hour to once a day.

Advice to the patient centered on the following:

1.   Reducing stress, anxiety, and worry.

2.   Maintaining bone strengthening exercises.

3.   Eating balanced, nutritious meals; reducing overconsumption of raw cold food, salads, frozen yogurt, and spoiled foods.

4.   Reduction/elimination of alcohol and late-night entertainment.

5.   Receiving acupuncture supplemented with auricular acupuncture, and taking herbs.

Specifically, I put her on a course of Fem-Estro, Cal-Apatite, and Recovery of Youth Tablets. Prior to selecting these, she had had poor results with *Liu Wei Di Huang Wan* (*Six Gentlemen Tea*) and Placenta Restorative Tablets. The first one produced lots of gas, commonly due to the *Yin* nature of the rehmannia root and her preexisting Spleen *Qi* deficiency. The second one made her itchy, which was perhaps an allergic reaction to the human placenta, another person's protein.

Chapter 18

Six Division Treatments, Three Paradigms of Treatment

Learning Objectives

Highly underutilized categories of points in the point classification system are the *Xi* (cleft) points. These points are very useful in the treatment of disease, especially for pain, which is a component of many illnesses. Additionally, few points are needed to address pain, sometimes as few as one, and this is helpful as people in pain do not like more discomfort that needles can evoke. The Six Division framework presented herein is not well known in contrast to its more popular use of explaining the progression of wind-cold pathogens into the body. By studying this chapter the practitioner will learn how to use these points in clinical practice in a new way with elegance and efficacy.

In the treatment of acute conditions, whether internal or musculoskeletal, practitioners strive to choose points whose therapeutic effectiveness has been established. Such options may fall into any category of points in the point classification system. One group of points that possesses unique functions for acute conditions where pain is a component is the *Xi* (cleft) points.

By definition, *Xi* (cleft) points are points of accumulation or blockage. They are considered reflex points of the organ–meridian complex; that is, their tenderness indicates problems in those meridians. They exhibit spontaneous or passive characteristics meaning pain or reaction when there is a blockage or accumulation in the corresponding organ–meridian complex.

An interesting approach to the treatment of painful conditions is the use of the Six Division framework as energetic layers to treat these problems. In this system, the use of the *Xi* (cleft) points of the meridians, paired together in Six Division framework, are the points employed. This treatment strategy reflects the Chinese cosmological view of "as above, so below." This expression means that both the organ–meridian complex impaired above, that is in the upper part of the body, and the corresponding complex below, the lower part of the body, will tend to be affected in acute conditions because of their Six Division coupling. This treatment strategy illustrates how to use the organ–meridian complexes paired in the Six Divisions with the traditional use of *Xi* (cleft) points as points of accumulation or blockage. Table 18.1, The Six Divisions, Associated *Xi* (cleft) Points, and the Side of the Body to Needle, instructs the practitioner on how to use them.

Table 18.1. The Six Divisions, Associated *Xi* (Cleft) Points, and the Side of the Body to Needle

Division	*Xi* (Cleft) Points	Side of the Body
Taiyang (SI/BL)	SI 6 (*Yanglao*) BL 63 (*Jinmen*)	Left Left
Shaoyang (TB/GB)	TB 7 (*Huizong*) GB 36 (*Waiqiu*)	Right Left
Yangming (ST/LI)	LI 7 (*Wenliu*) ST 34 (*Liangqiu*)	Right Right
Taiyin (LU/SP)	LU 6 (*Kongzui*) SP 8 (*Diji*)	Right Right
Jueyin (LR/PC)	LR 6 (*Zhongdu*) PC 4 (*Ximen*)	Left Left
Shaoyin (KI/HT)	HT 6 (*Yinxi*) KI 5 (*Shuiquan*)	Left Right and/or Left

A specific clinical example of an internal problem in which this strategy could be used would be with a patient who presents with an acute case of daytime asthma. There is tightness of the chest and shortness of breath with more difficulty on the exhale, wheezing due to phlegm, cough, spontaneous tenderness at LU 1 (*Zhongfu*), and a slippery Lung pulse. It is apparent that the Lung is the affected organ. In this case, the *Xi* (cleft) point of the Lung, Lung 6 (*Kongzui*), located in the upper *Jiao*, combined with the Xi (cleft) point of the Spleen, SP 8 (*Diji*), located in the lower *Jiao*, is chosen.

In the Six Division protocol unilateral needling is employed. Needle technique involves applying a dispersion technique to both *Xi* (cleft) points. The reason a dispersion technique is employed is to break up the accumulation or blockage in the Lungs as indicated by the phlegm and the tightness of the chest. There is no need for bilateral needling in many dispersion techniques because the needle technique should be strong and compensates for the use of two needles since meridians are connected on both sides In this case, Lung 6 (*Kongzhui*) and Spleen 8 (*Diji*) are needled on the right-hand side because the energetics of the Lung and Spleen are primarily right-sided as summarized in Table 16.7, A Historical Comparison of Various Pulse Diagnosis Systems, found in Chapter 16 and illustrated in Figure 18.1, Energy Crosses. Unilateral needling is based upon commonly accepted pulse assignments. In this case needling is performed unilaterally and all on the right side, although this would not be the case for all of the *Xi* (cleft) points, which can be seen when the pulse assignment chart is consulted.

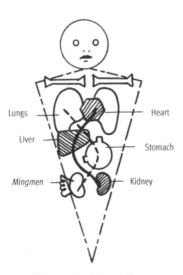

Figure 18.1: Energy Crosses

Needle technique is matched with the treatment plan, that is, we should apply strong dispersion techniques to the accumulation points. Needles need not be retained. An in-and-out technique with appropriate dispersion is all that is required. These points may either be used alone or as the skeletal basis of a treatment that addresses the major complaint. Some representative resolutions of disorders are listed here that employ the Six Division framework when the appropriate division is chosen.

- SI/BL: Increased range of neck and shoulder motion

- SI/BL: In cases of acute lumbar pain, immediate decrease of pain, area felt warmer, less clenching and stiffness

- TB/GB: Pain in the shoulder, hip, elbow, scapula, sacrum and shoulder—the most effective treatment the patient had in 5 yrs.

- SI/BL: Scapular and spine tenderness reduced

- SI/BL: Stiffness in arms, legs, and lumbar area felt better and lighter, standing more erect!

- LU/SP: Wind-cold invasion, occipital pain and stiffness reduced and felt like cold was leaving the body

Another example that involves the Lung/Spleen pair would be a case of acute dysmenorrhea, where the etiology of the painful period is stagnation due to *Blood* deficiency. Spleen 8 (*Diji*), the *Xi* (cleft) point, is chosen because of the accumulation or blockage that the painful period represents. In this case, the Spleen is failing to control the *Blood*. Not enough *Blood* is being produced and in turn this deficit is leading to stagnation. According to the Six Division model of "as above, so below," Lung 6 (*Kongzui*), the paired *Xi* (cleft) point, is selected. Table 18.2, Common Acute Clinical Conditions, Their Corresponding Six Division Level, *Xi* (Cleft) Points, and Supplementary Points, shows how to use them. Some commonly used supplementary points, to be added according to signs and symptoms after the *Xi* (cleft) point are needled and their effect evaluated, are also included.

Table 18.2. Common Acute Clinical Conditions, Their Corresponding Six Division Level, *Xi* (Cleft) Points, and Supplementary Points

Condition	Six Division Level and *Xi* (Cleft) Points	Supplementary Points
Acute Liver problems, menstrual problems	*Jueyin*: PC 4 (*Ximen*), LR 6 (*Zhongdu*)	LR 5 (*Ligou*)
Acute lumbago, declining eyesight in the elderly	*Taiyang*: SI 6 (*Yanglao*), BL 63 (*Jinmen*)	BL 1 (*Jingming*)
Acute menstrual problems (dysmenorrhea) or those due to *Qi* and *Blood* stagnation	*Taiyin*: LU 6 (*Kongzui*), SP 8 (*Diji*)	SP 10 (*Xuehai*)
Any blockage	*Shaoyang*: TE 7 (*Huizong*), GB 36 (*Wauqui*)	PC 6 (*Neiguan*)
Bleeding anywhere	*Taiyin*: LU 6 (*Kongzui*), SP 8 (*Diji*)	-
Chest pain, obesity, and heart disease	*Jueyin*: PC 4 (*Ximen*), LR 6 (*Zhongdu*)	KI 9 (*Zhubin*)
Hysteria, angina	*Shaoyin*: HT 6 (*Xinxi*), KI 5 (*Shuiquan*)	KI 9 (*Zhubin*)
Infantile convulsion	*Taiyang*: SI 6 (*Yanglao*), BL 63 (*Jinmen*)	KI 1 (*Yongquan*)
Mastitis	Yangming: LI 7 (*Wenliu*), ST 34 (*Linagqui*)	Ear: Liver, endocrine, mammary glands, *Shenmen*
Prostatitis	*Shaoyin*: HT 6 (*Xinxi*), KI 5 (*Shuiquan*)	CV 3 (*Zhongji*) BL 62 (*Shenmai*)
Rage	*Shaoyang*: TB 7 (*Huizong*), GB 36 (*Waiqui*)	-
Uterine hemorrhage (life threatening)	*Taiyin*: LU 6 (*Kongzui*), SP 8 (*Diji*)	SP 1 (*Yinbai*) LR 1 (*Dadun*)

If the patient's problem is musculoskeletal such as neck pain, back pain, or others, the treatment can be more efficacious if the patient mobilizes the affected area when one point is retained. This motion serves to work with the activation of the acupuncture point and consolidates the treatment. An example of this is offered in Case 9.

The Six Division framework is probably better known for use in other contexts. *The Shang Han Lun* (*Treatise of Cold-Induced Disorders*) outlines the progression of symptoms of a wind-cold or cold pathogen that has invaded the body and how those signs and symptoms change as the pathogen makes its way through these various energetic layers (Kaptchuk 1983). French acupuncturist Yves Requena explains the classical Chinese use of the Six Division paradigm to extrapolate on various personality/constitutional types that correspond to these energetic zones. More information on these approaches can be found by consulting the reference section (Requena 1989). The system described in this chapter represents another classical Chinese use of the Six Division model, an elegant, understated treatment strategy that yields dramatic and effective results when appropriately selected.

An interesting clinical adaptation of the use of *Xi* (cleft) points applies to the treatment of cancerous pain (Wenbing and Zhang 2000). Sometimes as practitioners who have cancer patients we need to address their pain and again the *Xi* (cleft) points rise to the fore as the points of choice.

Summary

The Six Division framework is one of the most highly underutilized and most efficient treatment plans in the treatment of pain. In fact it may even be unknown. Case 9 illustrates the use of the Six Division framework for a common clinical condition, backache. It is a powerful demonstration of how to select points for treatment based upon the classical energetics of the points, in this case *Xi* (cleft) points.

CASE 9: SIX DIVISIONS: AN ENERGETIC, PHILOSOPHICAL MODEL FOR PAIN AND BLOCKAGE IN THE TREATMENT OF BACK PAIN

The patient was a thirty-nine-year-old male who was experiencing an acute case of lumbago from trauma to the back. This condition was brought about by vigorous exercise. He had not worked out strenuously in a long time and had a history of minor episodes of back strain usually brought on by lifting heavy objects, a common cause of acute lumbago.

For this patient, the usual treatment after such an injury would be rest, hot baths with relaxing bath salts, the application of Chinese liniments and bruise plasters, and ibuprofen, all of which would give some relief for a certain time. On this particular occasion, the back strain was quite severe and six weeks later he still had not recovered. He sought the assistance of an acupuncturist.

In this particular case, I opted to use the Six Division framework. I chose SI 6 (*Yanglao*) and BL 63 (*Jinmen*), the *Xi* (cleft) points that specifically treat acute lumbago. SI 6 (*Yanglao*), in the upper part of the body, was needled first on the left side. The point was needled with a thick needle, #28, 30mm and a strong stimulus, proximally in the direction of the flow of the meridian with a dispersive technique. The patient felt strong energy go up his arm. At the same time the patient was instructed to mobilize his back by standing and swaying to activate the affected area. His back immediately felt better even though he had endured six weeks of pain that ranged from immobilizing to residual discomfort.

To strengthen the effect, BL 63 (*Jinmen*), the corresponding *Xi* (cleft) point, was also needled on the left side against the flow of energy in the meridian. However, the effect was not as strong as with SI 6 (*Yanglao*) because SI 6 (*Yanglao*) had acted so well. The needles were retained only for the amount of time it took to achieve the desired needle sensation and to note the improvement. After this treatment the patient said that his back was fine.

Chapter 19

Heat Differentiations

Learning Objectives

The purpose of this chapter is to clarify for the practitioner the types of heat found in the human body. Clinically, especially with students, the etiology of heat is misunderstood and thus treated incorrectly. Additionally there is a variety of heat due to *Qi* deficiency that is not recognized by even experienced practitioners. These important differentiations are discussed herein.

TRUE HEAT AND *YIN* DEFICIENCY HEAT

As we recall, there are two types of heat, true heat and false heat. This may sound elemental and it is, but rudimentary principles are not necessarily easy to understand and this differentiation and its concomitant treatment plan is frequently missing in clinic and has serious consequences so a review is worthwhile.

True heat is often called real, excessive, solid, and replete heat caused by invasion of pathogenic factors like exogenous pathogenic heat or summer heat, pathogens that stagnate and turn to heat, or heat in the organs. True heat can come from organs that are hot through the introduction of hot natured foods and drinks like excess spices, chile, alcohol, red meat, and sugar. In the clinical arena, true heat manifests as a red tongue with a yellow coat and perhaps dry. The pulse is rapid and excessive, the face and/or neck red, and the voice is loud and sonorous. Anger may be present as well as other signs of true heat such as thirst. The aim of treatment is to reduce or clear the heat. Moxibustion in this scenario is contraindicated.

False heat is not real heat. It is called *Yin* deficient heat. It looks like heat, that is, there are heat manifestations, but its origin is deficiency of *Yin*. What looks like heat is true *Yang*. False heat manifestations include a thin, red tongue with little or no fur, a weak, thin, fast pulse, and red cheeks in the afternoon, a thin body, night sweats, and perhaps irritability. The treatment plan is to nourish the *Yin*. This can be done with all the things that nourish *Yin* such as acupuncture points that are needled that tonify *Yin* or with herbs. However, we need to note that there are three types of *Yin* deficiency: *Yin* deficiency, *Yin* deficiency with heat, and *Yin* deficiency with fire.

Yin deficiency can be measured on a continuum. *Yin* deficiency does not have heat signs, for instance, the person is thin, has a thin pulse, or a thin tongue. *Yin* deficiency with heat is accompanied by heat such as a thin, red tongue, a thin fast pulse, thirst with small sips, and malar flush. *Yin* deficiency with fire has more virulent heat symptoms that we call fire such as a deep red tongue with thorns, night sweats, mouth sores, and other signs of hyperactivity of fire.

Note that moxibustion is only contraindicated in *Yin* deficiency with heat or fire but not for *Yin* deficiency. In fact, the classics point out that for all cases of deficiency of *Qi*, *Blood*, *Yin*, or *Yang*, moxibustion is essential. The *Miraculous Pivot* maintains, "Deficiency of both Yin and Yang should be treated with moxa" (Cheng 1999, p.361). The *Yin* meridians carry not only *Jing* fluid but also fire to help them in their function of nourishing and moistening. So if using moxa in *Yin* deficiency cases, monitor the patient closely for signs of heat aggravation such as fever, restlessness, and insomnia, and use small moxa modalities such as thread moxas, tiger thermie, or other small quantities of moxa so that the *Yin* deficiency does not turn into *Yin* deficiency with heat.

Yin deficiency does increase with age. By the time one is in their 40's the *Yin* is half consumed especially the *Yin* of the Kidney. We can see that decline in the *Qi* cycle for men and women so that perspective should be helpful in guiding your diagnosis.

QI DEFICIENCY HEAT

Herein we take a look at a mysterious yet logical etiology of heat that oftentimes is misdiagnosed, that is, heat due to *Qi* deficiency. As the name points out, *Qi* deficiency heat or fire if stronger has as its origin *Qi* deficiency. In order to understand the nature of this heat, we have to understand its etiology. Because the treatment principle is correlated with the diagnosis we need to know where the heat comes from in order to correctly treat this condition.

The problem with *Qi* deficiency, apart from any deficiency manifestation, is that it may stagnate. For the most part stagnation turns to heat due to the lack of movement combined with the underlying human substrate of our nature as warm-blooded animals. Relatively speaking, as moving, sentient, growing organisms we are more *Yang* than *Yin*, about 3/5 to 2/5 respectively. When the *Qi* that is stagnant adapts to our underlying *Yang* terrain it turns to heat. This is true of all of the six stagnations called *Liu yu*: *Qi*, *Blood*, Damp/Phlegm, Heat, Cold, and Food.

If the heat is arising out of *Qi* deficiency leading to *Qi* stagnation manifesting as heat, our aim of treatment is to tonify the *Qi*, but slowly and carefully so as not to cause heat exacerbation. As we know, the organ most prone to stagnation is the Liver and it is the job of the Liver to promote the free flowingness of *Qi* and *Blood* throughout the organism. We do not talk about Liver *Qi* deficiency as a *Zang-fu* syndrome although we do have Liver *Blood* deficiency as a syndrome. Since the *Qi* is the commander of the *Blood* this is the approach rather than to tonify Liver *Qi*, which we do not speak of. When the Liver *Qi* stagnates due to *Qi* deficiency (but not of the Liver), or *Blood* stagnation of the Liver, we may get heat. The heat can occur with movement, as simple as turning over in bed in the night when the *Blood* returns to the Liver and builds up as we are reclining. This movement may cause hot flashes. Or the heat may occur as a result of exertion like exercise as the *Qi* stagnation is freed up via that movement.

The Liver derives its *Qi* from the Lung via the *Ko* (control cycle), and also from the *Yang* of the Kidney, so healthy Lung and Kidney functioning is important. Remember that the Lung is the Master of the *Qi* but if the Lung is weak, how can we strengthen the Lung? Remember a Five Element strategy: When an element is deficient, tonify the mother. The Mother of Lungs is the Spleen. Strengthening Spleen *Qi* is the key to tonifying the Lung *Qi*. This will also tonify the Kidney *Yang* and thusly move stagnant Liver *Qi* and the heat stasis.

There are numerous approaches to do this, for instance exercises that strengthen the muscles that belong to the Spleen build *Qi* and move *Blood*. Tonifying herbs that tonify Spleen *Qi* and move *Blood* and clear some heat are useful. Diets that strengthen Spleen *Qi* versus Damp foods that weaken it also help. This three-pronged lifestyle approach will produce faster results. If properly diagnosed and treated, heat manifestations should immediately abate in frequency, duration, and intensity and over a 2–3 month period be under control and on the way to resolution as long as healthy lifestyle practices continue. Herbs and foods that also augment *Yin* are also helpful as *Yin* can assist the *Qi* in moving, and *Yin* helps to create more *Blood*, the other more liquid side so to speak of *Qi*. Ten Needle Technique described in Chapter 12 is a great treatment strategy for tonifying *Qi*, *Blood*, *Yin*, and *Yang*. For clinical convenience Table 19.1, The Differentiation of Heat, summarizes the etiology, clinical manifestations, and treatment principles when heat is present.

Table 19.1. The Differentiation of Heat

Diagnosis	Causative Factor	Clinical Manifestations	Treatment
Excess heat/fire	Invasion of exogenous heat pathogens, i.e. heat, summer heat, wind heat True organ heat, i.e. heat in the Stomach	Red face, red tongue, rapid full pulse May be sweating, thirst, restlessness, anxiety, palpitations, insomnia, red eyes, hunger	Clear excess heat
Yin deficiency heat or fire	Heat or fire due to *Yin* deficiency. This is false heat meaning the heat is a reflection of the true *Yang*	Malar flush, thin rapid pulse, red tongue, no coat, five palm heat, night sweats	Subdue *Yin* heat or fire by nourishing the *Yin*
Qi deficiency heat	Heat due to *Qi* deficiency of the Spleen, Lung and Kidney May be *Blood* deficiency as well	Heat generated by movement or exertion or produced through Liver stasis such as daytime sweat, heat sensations, night sweats and hot flashes	Tonify Spleen *Qi*, to tonify Lung *Qi* and Kidney *Yang* to move Liver *Qi* stagnation

Summary ——————————————

The differentiation of heat is critical to the health of your patient. It is important to understand its etiology and concomitant treatment principle.

Chapter 20

A Synopsis of Bloodletting Techniques

Learning Objectives

Bleeding is a simple and efficacious treatment modality that is the method of choice for certain clinical conditions and disease differentiations. The practitioner should learn these clinical scenarios and be able to bleed with skill and success.

Included in the repertoire of the Nine Ancient Needles expounded upon in the *Lingshu* was the use of the three-edge needle, a needle with a large puncture point. The modern three-edge needle is derived from this early type. It is obvious from inspecting the modern three-edge needle that the tip does not have the usual point configuration of filiform needles. Rather, it has a triangular head designed to make a larger hole in the skin for bloodletting. Because many commercial bleeding needles are of such poor quality that their tips are jagged and can actually damage tissue, practitioners frequently substitute medical lancets for the same purpose. Ordinary acupuncture needles can also be used and in this case, a large gauge needle such as a #28 or #30 gauge, 15mm needle should be selected.

The three-edge needle was conceived to treat clinical conditions through the following three therapeutic aims:

1. To promote the smooth flow of *Qi* and *Blood* in the meridians or tissues by stimulating the channel.

2. To dispel *Blood* stasis and activate *Qi* and *Blood* by promoting its unobstructed flow.

3. To drain heat or fire.

Clinical conditions that are manifestations of these disorders will be discussed later in this chapter.

The anatomical locations of most of the points that are bled are relatively shallow places such as superficial blood vessels. Other commonly bled points include ear points, scalp points, and *Jing* (well) points that are located close to the surface. *Jing* (well) points lend themselves to bleeding not only because of their superficial location but also because of their inherent energy as discussed in Chapter 8. As a reminder, as the most distal points on a meridian, furthest away from the center of energy in the body, *Jing* (well) points are sites where the energy of a meridian is like water filling a well. The energy is just starting to appear and bubble. From a Five Element point of view, the use of these points is particularly appropriate for the Spring season as well as the "Spring" of a disease, that is, the early, acute stages of a disorder. At the nexus of the *Jing* (well) points, the qualities of *Yin* and *Yang* are less differentiated and tend to merge. Hence they are especially beneficial in effecting a rapid transformation of energy from *Yang* to *Yin* or *Yin* to *Yang*. Thus these points are useful for balancing, for changing polarity, and for expelling fullness in the organs.

TYPES OF BLEEDING

The most common form of manipulation of the bloodletting needle is the spot pricking or collateral pricking technique. Collaterals refer to the meridians and vessels. Most points, such as *Jing* (well) points, are punctured in this manner. Prior to inserting the needle, the point should be massaged or squeezed and secured with the nondominant hand to cause slight venous pooling so that when the needle is inserted blood will be released. After the skin is pricked and a small puncture is made so that blood is extracted, a clean cotton ball should be applied to the site and pressed firmly to absorb the droplets and stop the bleeding. An adhesive bandage should also be put over the puncture site for a short amount of time to prevent any infection and to stop any further bleeding.

A second technique involves making tiny pinprick motions to the affected area until blood is released. This method is referred to as the clumping or area pricking method. This technique is suitable for reddened skin tissue, bruising, and extravasation, or other overt signs of *Blood* stagnation. After the punctures have been made, the epidermis should be squeezed to obtain more blood. Following the escape of the *Blood*, it should be absorbed with a cotton ball and then covered with an adhesive bandage, or antiseptic solution, again to prevent infection.

Thirdly, in the pinching method, pinching the skin with the nondominant hand, and pricking the affected area with the bleeding needle to induce bleeding can facilitate bloodletting. Other devices such as the plum blossom needle, also called a Seven Star or cutaneous needle, a regular acupuncture needle, or the Japanese *shoni-shin* needle can be employed to stimulate a large area so that superficial bleeding occurs.

In bleeding techniques, speed is essential in puncturing the point to reduce sustained contact with the free nerve endings. The depth of insertion for these points is very shallow ranging between .05 and .1 *cun*.

All contraindications for needling apply in bloodletting. If the patient has generalized weakness, anemia, a hypotensive condition, hemorrhagic disease, or is pregnant or recently delivered, bloodletting should not be used. The course of treatment varies from one treatment or until the condition is rectified. Treat once per day or on alternate days. If the patient bleeds a lot, treat one to two times per week or not at all.

A survey of the indications of the acupuncture points of the body reveals that numerous points lend themselves to bleeding, and indeed in the clinical conditions listed in Table 20.1, The Bleeding Needle: Points to Needle for Specific Clinical Conditions, bleeding is the method of choice to bring about the desired therapeutic result. However, the indications are by no means exhaustive. Inflammation, with its characteristic signs of redness, swelling, heat, and pain is well treated through this method. For example, for a swollen ankle, a plum blossom needle can be used. This treatment is generally quite painful when administered but is also unsurpassed in activating the flow of *Qi* and *Blood* to the affected area. The prognosis is greatly enhanced and the resolution is accelerated by this technique. Red, swollen, painful arthritis, neurodermatitis, allergic dermatitis, rhinitis, headache, erysipelas, lymphatitis, and hemorrhoids can also be treated in this way.

Table 20.1. The Bleeding Needle: Points to Needle for Specific Clinical Conditions

Points	Conditions
LU 11 (*Shaoshang*)	Sore throat of the excess type, i.e., exogenous invasion, tonsillitis, stuffiness and pain in chest, asthmatic breathing, stomachache, frontal shoulder pain
LI 1 (*Shangyang*)	Toothache, sore throat, nasal obstruction, tinnitus, frontal headache, stomachache, shoulder pain
ST 8 (*Touwei*)	Pain and redness in eyes
HT 9 (*Shaochong*)	Febrile diseases, stuffiness and pain in the chest, palpitations, angina pectoris, insomnia, headache, tinnitus, shoulder pain, back pain, heart attack
SI 1 (*Shaoze*)	Febrile diseases, breast disorders, breast tenderness
BL 2 (*Zhanzhu*)	Wind-heat in the eyes, acute conjunctivitis, sinus pressure and headache
BL 40 (*Weizhong*)	Back pain, acute lumbar sprain, multiple furuncles and swelling, sunstroke, leg pain
BL 67 (*Zhiyin*)	Back pain on Bladder channel
PC 3 (*Quze*)	Febrile disease, acute vomiting
PC 9 (*Zhongjong*)	Coma, unconsciousness, stuffiness and pain in chest, palpitations, angina, insomnia, Stomach problems, pain in Liver region
TB 1 (*Guanchong*)	Tinnitus, migraine, sore throat, shoulder pain, back pain, pain in the chest and hypochondriac region, hepatic distending pain
LR 1 (*Dadun*)	Irritability, red eyes, red face, genital pain, purple toes
GV 4 (*Mingmen*)	Lumbago
GV 14 (*Dazhui*) and its Huatoujiajis*	Lung heat (excess), febrile disease, pneumonia
GV 20 (*Baihui*)	Stiff neck
GV 26 (*Shuigou*)	Lumbago

EXTRA POINTS	
Taiyang	Acute conjunctivitis, hypertension
Yintang	Headache
Erjian (ear apex)	Acute conjunctivitis, spasms, high fever caused by toxicity, wind, heat, Liver *Yang* rising
Jinjin and *Yuyue* (veins under tongue)	Pernicious vomiting, aphasia
Shixuan (tips of fingers)	Coma, epilepsy, infantile convulsions, sunstroke
Sifeng (midpoint of interphalangeal joints of all fingers except thumb)	Digestive disorders in children (prick when purple; white fluid may come out)
Baxie (junction of margin of webs of fingers)	Spasm and contracture of the fingers (pathologic fluid may come out)
Local points	Varicose veins, spider veins, phlebitis
Jing (well) points	Numbness, stroke, febrile disease, resuscitation
COMBINATIONS	
LI 4 (*Hegu*), LI 11 (*Quchi*)	Numbness
ST 36 (*Zusanli*), GV 26 (*Shuigou*), PC 3 (*Quze*), BL 40 (*Weizhong*), PC 6 (*Neiguan*), *Jing* (well) points	Hypertension
BL 40 (*Weizhong*), LU 5 (*Chize*), ST 44 (Neiting), PC 3 (*Quze*)	Sunstroke, acute gastroenteritis, food poisoning
Luo points	For acute local swelling

*The *Huatoujiaji* points mentioned here are a group of points on both sides of the spinal column .5 *cun* lateral borders of each spinous process from the first thoracic vertebra to the fifth lumbar vertebra

Some common reactions to bleeding are provided for an appreciation of bloodletting as a modality:

- Acute ankle injury—immediate alleviation of pain

- Hip and low back pain—felt amazing

- Shoulder pain—pain 90% better and normal range of motion, could move arm without pain, improved abduction

- Acute burning epigastric pain—pain gone

- Anxiety and insomnia—less edgy

- Very sore throat—immediate relief

THE TREATMENT OF *BLOOD* STASIS WITH BLEEDING TECHNIQUES

We have seen that bleeding techniques are invaluable in the treatment of *Blood* stasis because of their ability to promote the free flow of *Qi* and *Blood*, to disperse *Blood* stasis, and to eliminate heat or fire. A rather serious manifestation of *Blood* stasis is an accumulation of *Blood* at the base of the occiput that can occur in cases of high blood pressure and/or as an early sign of stroke. It resembles a large bruise or birthmark and ranges in color from red to dark purple.

Anatomically, the occiput is predisposed to energetic blockages because it is a physical protuberance. *Qi* stagnation in the form of neck tension, subluxated vertebrae, and arthritic bone deformities are common manifestations of this predisposition. When *Blood* stagnation develops in this area, it is an unfavorable condition that needs to be treated immediately with the modality of choice, bloodletting.

As a prestroke manifestation, the patient generally has a history of hypertension or minimally labile blood pressure, that is, the person's blood pressure changes in response to environmental stimuli. Because it appears at the base of the skull, usually in the GB 20 (*Fengchi*) area, patients are generally not aware of the presence of the extravasated *Blood* because they cannot see it. *Blood* stasis, a physical blockage, represents a potential embolism and/or a blockage that can lead to the creation of internal wind, which can be a precipitating factor in the development of stroke. The stasis must be dispelled to avert such a dangerous situation.

Other signs and symptoms will prompt the skilled practitioner to examine this area. If the patient is simultaneously noting tongue and facial discomfort, it indicates that the Heart is involved and that there is a lack of *Blood* flow to the face. I know of no sources that state, "If the tongue feels 'weird,' there is Heart involvement." However, the tongue as the sprout of the Heart suggests some connection, and my clinical experience verifies this. These symptoms include severe emotional distress, an odd sensation in the tongue, and facial numbness on the side where the ecchymosis is present. In addition, the patient may have a deviated tongue, an early sign of wind stroke. If the patient mentions the tongue and facial sensations, the practitioner should immediately inspect the neck and treat it if the *Blood* stasis is present, but these are late stages of high blood pressure. I recommend as part of the physical exam to inspect the occipital area and treat if early signs of *Blood* stasis are present.

Apart from cases of hypertension, other patients with labile blood pressure may also develop *Blood* stasis in situations of emotional distress. Usually, they are aware of something going on in the occipital area because the skin becomes unbearably itchy there. Inspection by the practitioner reveals the characteristic *Blood* stagnation mark. Although any of the above methods can be used to invigorate the smooth flow of *Qi* and *Blood* and thus disperse the *Blood* stagnation, the *shoni-shin* needle or plum blossom needle is practical because the patient can keep the needle for self-treatment. In addition, the opposite end of the *shoni-shin* needle has a scraping edge that can also be used by the patient to move the *Qi* and *Blood* and relieve itchiness without piercing the skin, similar to the modality of *Gwa Sha*. The needle many be hard to find for purchase outside of Japan, in which case use a plum blossom needle.

Under these conditions it is imperative to disperse the *Blood* stasis. We can do this with any number of tools that can produce bloodletting, such as the plum blossom needle, the tri-edge needle, a regular acupuncture needle, or *shoni-shin* needle. How to use each of these instruments is summarized in Table 20.2, Bloodletting Techniques for *Blood* Stasis Patterns in the Occipital Area.

Table 20.2. Bloodletting Techniques for *Blood*
Stasis Patterns in the Occipital Area

Instrument	Method
Plum blossom needle	Quickly and vigorously tap the skin of the affected area so that a slight amount of blood is released. Carefully absorb the blood with a sterile piece of gauze and dispose of it properly. Re-usable or disposable plum blossom needles may be used. Sterilize or dispose of properly
Bleeding needle or lancet	With a specialized bleeding needle (tri-edge needle) repeatedly pierce the affected area. If this needle or a medical lancet is used, more blood will be extracted because of the size of the needle tip. Use the same quick and vigorous insertion technique, but pierce less frequently over the same skin area if you want less bleeding
Filiform needle	Quickly and vigorously pierce the affected area. Repeatedly release small droplets of blood as with the plum blossom and tri-edge needle techniques. Use a #28 or #30 gauge needle. Some patients tolerate the repeated insertion of this needle better than the piercing done by the plum blossom needle that can be aggravating because of the number of needles in its head. It is also less painful than a lancet or a tri-edge needle because of its smaller tip. This is my preferred method of bloodletting
Shoni-shin needle	This small plastic pediatric needle can also be substituted for any of the previous techniques. The clinical utility of this needle, apart from its effectiveness, is that it is plastic and disposable, whereas the reusable plum blossom needle needs to be sterilized before reuse, if used on different patients. Also, the patients can keep the needle and treat themselves
	Dispose of the plum blossom needle in a biohazard container

Only draw a small amount of blood with these techniques; the droplets may actually be very small, but they should be present and make the breakup and invigoration of *Qi* and *Blood* obvious. Although this is a highly specific treatment for a unique clinical condition and is very beneficial for the patient, the practitioner should not risk her or his own health by exposure to blood-borne pathogens. Follow Occupational, Safety, and Health Administration (OSHA) guidelines. As in all cases of pricking, clean needle technique must be employed. Needles must be sterile, and it is highly advisable for the practitioner to wear a double pair of gloves. Goggles as well as a facial mask are also recommended to protect the practitioner from the aerosolized blood that can be generated by a vigorous bloodletting style in the case of plum blossom usage. Use your professional judgment.

Cases 10 and 11 illustrate the clinical use of bloodletting techniques.

CASE 10: *BLOOD* STASIS PATTERNS IN THE OCCIPITAL REGION

The patient was a seventy-four-year-old female with many serious health problems. She sought acupuncture treatment primarily for the effects of knee surgery and a car accident. She had shooting pains in her thighs and left big toe. Other health problems included high blood pressure, arthritis, a personal history of heart attack, and extreme emotional agitation from family problems. There were many other complaints that unfolded weekly from this friendly and talkative patient. At the time of the initial intake, I noticed that the tongue was grossly enlarged and deviated. Regardless of how the patient was doing from week to week, this fact always concerned me.

The patient was inconsistent in taking her high blood pressure medication because of its cost at that time of $1.80 per day. I could not convince her of the danger of this practice and even had a medical doctor explain to her the seriousness of not taking her medication regularly, but to no avail.

The patient received acupuncture treatments twice a week and responded favorably. Within five months, many of her problems were resolved as well as most symptoms related to the major complaint. However, there were still symptoms that I was particularly concerned about. These included dizziness, cold sweats, a weak quivery voice, armpit pain, and numbness of the left arm, fatigue, and insomnia. In addition, the patient reported that her tongue felt swollen and that it burned. She could feel her heart on the left side, her left arm hurt, she was tired, and had "heartburn." Her left eye was hard to close and felt heavy. She also had occasional flashes in her head and her blood pressure remained consistently high. I insisted that she see her heart specialist immediately, but she refused because of the cost of tests, time constraints, and a feeling of lack of rapport and trust with the specialists.

Acupuncture treatment temporarily brought her blood pressure down and the head flashes stopped. The patient finally saw her cardiologist after I made an appointment for her. The blood pressure continued to stay elevated, she felt pressure on the left side of the head, her lips felt numb, and her eyes were blurry. These symptoms suggested an imminent heart attack or stroke. At this point, I inspected the base of the skull and saw the characteristic *Blood* stasis hematoma.

I immediately explained the plum blossom bloodletting technique to the patient and began to treat the affected area. Within seconds the patient reported that the "weird" feeling in her tongue was diminishing. After a few minutes of therapy the facial numbness and heaviness were gone. The effects of this treatment lasted for about three weeks.

One month later the patient reported many serious symptoms: four nights of insomnia due to palpitations, shortness of breath made worse by laying down, feeling her heart pound in her ears, head distention, generalized stiffness on the left side, her mouth feeling funny, a feeling of a "dead" spot on the right side of her face, "heartburn," sleeping in the day, swollen feet, numbness of the arms and legs, feeling like she weighed "500 pounds," and a bitter taste in the mouth. She had a deep red tongue and a fast pulse. Also, her high blood pressure, for which she was not taking her medication, continued.

Treatment with the plum blossom needle helped diminish the numbness, heaviness, and weird feelings, however the patient was admonished to seek Western medical help. Two weeks later she admitted herself to the emergency room as she finally recognized the seriousness of her problem. She explained to the doctor that an acupuncturist had been treating her for heart attack/prestroke symptoms and he told her that the bloodletting treatment she received had probably prevented her from having a stroke. The easy sweat and tiredness with lack of exertion continued and further medical tests revealed low levels of oxygen in the blood.

Shortly thereafter the patient's insurance company would no longer pay for her acupuncture treatment since the major complaint of trauma related injuries were resolved. Even though I offered her unlimited free treatments, the patient had already run up bills that the insurance company would not pay when the emphasis in treatment changed, and her pride would not allow her to accept free treatment.

I cautioned her to take her medications and to see her cardiologist. I told her as well to call if she needed any further treatment that she thought I could offer her.

CASE 11: ADDITIONAL CASE OF *BLOOD* STASIS PATTERNS IN THE OCCIPITAL REGION

The patient was a thirty-five-year-old female with an acute complaint of unbearable scalp itchiness. She was applying a corticosteroid cream, which was recommended by a dermatologist. Also, she was using a Chinese liniment prescribed by a private practitioner. Neither solution was working.

One day in passing, she mentioned to me that these modalities were not helping and that she was desperate. At the same time, she was experiencing a series of family tragedies. In characteristic fashion, she was taking on and internalizing all these problems and she told me that she had not given herself the time to cry yet. She had tightness in the chest and throat, extreme grief, anger, and heightened irritability. Inspection of the patient confirmed that she had a tendency to hold things in. Her complexion was greenish-black with an underlying sallowness to it. Her blood pressure was generally low, but could become situationally labile.

Because I was going to see what I could do on an emergency basis, I used what I had gained from observation as well as minimal but focused questioning. When I asked to see where the itchiness was, the patient pointed to the base of the occiput in the GV 15 (*Yamen*), GV 16 (*Fengfu*), and GB 20 (*Fengchi*) area. I could clearly see the characteristic *Blood* stasis pattern.

I began repeatedly piercing the ecchymosis while the patient sat with her head bent forward onto a desk. Dark red-black blood began to emerge, and within one minute the patient reported that the unbearable itchiness that had plagued her for weeks was gone. To disperse the stasis I advised her to scratch the affected area with the comb-like edge of the *shoni-shin* needle if the itchiness recurred. I also told her to disperse the stasis and to apply *Zheng Gu Shui* to the affected area if the needle did not help to further invigorate the *Blood*. Shortly after the treatment, in less than an hour, the grief from her suppressed emotions began to be released and the problem was totally resolved.

COMMON USES OF THE PLUM BLOSSOM NEEDLE

Apart from conditions where bloodletting is desired, the plum blossom needle as a vehicle for facilitating the free flow of *Qi* and *Blood* can also be used. This section addresses some difficult-to-treat conditions where the plum blossom needle can be used effectively. These conditions include myopia and other eye problems, baldness, varicose veins, the common cold, constipation, migraines, and acute conjunctivitis. Other conditions include skin diseases, nervous system numbness, high blood pressure, headache, vertigo, and dizziness.

Table 20.3 outlines the clinical condition and the corresponding method of treatment to use with the plum blossom needle. Case 12 describes an effective application of this technique. A note of caution: Do not use the plum blossom needle on the face, ulcerations, or on weak patients.

Table 20.3. The Treatment of Common Clinical
Conditions with the Plum Blossom Needle

Condition	Treatment
Eye problems, such as myopia, lacrimation, and atrophy of the optic nerve	Plum blossom LI 14 (*Binao*), GB 37 (*Guangming*), *Taiyang*, and an extra point between the eyebrow and the eyeball, GB 20 (*Fengchi*) due to its relationship to the visual cortex in the occipital lobe, GV 14 (*Dazhui*), PC 6 (*Neiguan*) to regulate the *Qi* and *Blood* of the entire body. Also, as Master of the *Yinwei Mai* it brings energy to the eyes. ST 1 (*Chengqi*) and GB 1 (*Tonzilliao*). Supplement with the following auricular points for good effect: Eye 1, 2, 3, occiput, *Shenmen*, LR, ST, SP, KI
Baldness (especially an acute onset)	Tap heavily over the affected area, and then apply fresh ginger juice
Varicose veins*	Tap very lightly on the protruding veins; do not try to elicit blood. Use a zigzag motion along the veins and move from lower part of the leg and upward
Common cold	Tap along the medial Bladder lines, as well as along both sides of the nose
Constipation	Administer on the lower abdomen and on the back in the lumbar-sacral region
Migraine	Tap on the nape of the neck on the affected side, on PC 6 (*Neiguan*), TB 5 (*Waiguan*), and in the sacral region
Acute conjunctivitis	Tap in the area of the cervical vertebrae (C1–4), around the eyes, on GB 20 (*Fengchi*), *Taiyang*, and LI 4 (*Hegu*)

* The Chinese doctors I studied with differentiate varicose veins as a Kidney, not a Spleen problem, since it occurs in the lower *Jiao* and is generally accompanied by edema. Also, older people whose Kidney *Qi* declines tend to develop it

CASE 12: THE APPLICATION OF THE PLUM BLOSSOM NEEDLE IN THE TREATMENT OF HAIR LOSS

The patient was a forty-eight-year-old woman whose major complaint was hair loss. At the time she came to seek Chinese medical treatment the problem had been going on for six years. Since its onset she had lost about half of her hair, most of it from the right side. The problem had become more pronounced within the last year.

Her hair was coming out by the roots. Its texture was dry and the color was fading. The patient's scalp felt tight around the crown area and the tightness was worsened by stress. She felt pinpricking pain on the right side of her scalp and at the base of her skull, so much so that the pain woke her up at night. She also felt cold on that side of her head. Her hair was thin, particularly around the Gall Bladder and other *Yang* channels of the head. The patient presented with several other major complaints, many health problems, and subpathologies. In treating this chronic problem, it was important that the patient's major complaint not be isolated from the context of who she was, that is, from all of her health problems. However, without enumerating them all, the patient's root diagnosis was *Blood* deficiency leading to *Blood* stagnation.

The pattern of hair loss is clearly one of deficiency, specifically of the *Blood*. The hair is the extension of the *Blood* and the head hair belongs to the Kidney. All of her signs and symptoms including weak left superficial pulses and the pale, thin, dry tongue suggested a *Blood* deficiency.

There was some *Blood* stagnation in the head from the deficiency and this created the tight feeling over the crown area and the pinpricking sensation. The treatment principle was directed at tonifying the *Blood*, dispersing *Blood* stagnation, and tonifying the *Qi* of the Kidney. Many treatment modalities were selected for the patient, including plum blossom needling, moxa, acupuncture, herbal therapy, nutritional counseling, and exercise advice.

To address the major complaint, the plum blossom needle was selected as the tool of choice for the affected area followed by an application of fresh ginger juice. Even though the hair loss was a long-term problem, this strategy had the combined effect of dispersing stagnation as well as increasing circulation to the affected area. Moxibustion was administered in the form of the moxa box on the abdomen to tonify the internal deficiency that had manifested as *Blood* deficiency and internal cold. Acupuncture was selected to adjust the *Qi* and *Blood*. Herbs were chosen to build as well as move *Blood*. Dietary counseling was critical to compensate for a history of poor eating habits along with a vegetarian diet that together had further weakened the body's capacity to produce *Blood* and anchor the hair, so to speak. Exercise regimes were discussed to strengthen the *Qi* and *Blood* as well as move the stagnation.

The patient received treatment in the office three times a month for three months and then came back for a final treatment and a consultation two months later. The patient took herbs, tried to eat better, and administered the plum blossom technique on herself. After the first treatment, which included the plum blossom technique to the GV 20 (*Baihui*) and GB 20 (*Fengchi*) areas, the scalp tightness was reduced and her energy level was higher. Three weeks later she only experienced one night of pricking scalp pain and no scalp tightness, even though she had been extremely stressed. By her tenth and final treatment the hair loss had stopped, the pricking pain had abated, and there was almost no head tension. When head tension did develop the patient could always correlate it with stress that she was not managing. These results were maintained for three years without further treatment.

In my opinion, the success of this treatment, not only with regard to the major complaint but also to many of the patient's other serious health problems, was based on the recognition of the common denominator of all of her health problems. Excellent patient compliance and herbal therapy enhanced the effects. This is an interesting case of a *Blood* deficiency problem manifesting as hair loss that was well treated through augmenting the simple yet appropriate tool of the plum blossom needle.

GWA SHA: SCRAPING EVIL WETNESS

Supplementing the tapping and bleeding techniques designed to treat the manifestations of *Blood* stasis is another modality, that of *Gwa Sha*, a scraping mechanism. Although it is not technically a bleeding technique, its effects are so similar that I have included it here.

Gwa Sha, translated as "scraping evil wetness" or "scraping sand," can be used in two manifestations of evil wetness which is either stagnant *Blood*, or Dampness in the body as secondary pathological products, or both. In the case of *Blood* stagnation from an internal or miscellaneous origin, from *Qi* deficiency, retardation in the flow of *Qi* and *Blood*, trauma or injury, this scraping technique helps to activate the abnormal or obstructed flow of *Qi* and *Blood* in the joints and muscles.

Gwa Sha is useful for the following:

- Promoting the circulation of *Qi* and *Blood* as in the case of sprains

- Warming and dispelling cold as in the case of *Blood* stasis, asthma, and paralysis

- Removing excess as in facial paralysis

- Removing painful obstructions due to wind, cold, damp, and heat such as rheumatism of the joints

The scraping motion of *Gwa Sha* is executed with a firm-edged tool such as a pediatric scraping needle, the comb-like edge of the *shoni-shin* needle, or any other similar device. I prefer to use the firm edge of a Chinese soupspoon; it is not only aesthetic and comfortable in the hand but does the job well. Using a brisk, short, flicking action, the chosen apparatus is applied over the affected area in a simultaneous top-to-bottom and medial-to-lateral direction. This vigorous, superficial massage technique improves the circulation of *Qi* and *Blood* to the affected area. Parts of the body that are commonly treated with *Gwa Sha* include the neck, joints, legs, abdomen, back, and musculoskeletal regions. Because we are trying to move stagnation, this vigorous technique may result in bruising, tenderness, tiredness, or invigoration, and the patient should be informed of these possible side effects and/or sign a consent for *Gwa Sha* form.

For added result, *Gwa Sha* can be used in combination with appropriate acupuncture points. Liniments can also be used to move *Qi* and *Blood* and to clear the channels. Lubricating liniments such as Regal Oil, *Possum On*, Woodlock Oil, and *Wan Hua* can be applied to the skin prior to the *Gwa Sha* and the cupping. Apply an ample amount of the selected oil to the affected area and then administer the *Gwa Sha* technique. Apply less vigorously to patients with delicate skin or to those who bruise easily. Scrape the affected area once with each stroke, making your way from top to bottom. Repeat this procedure three to five times depending upon the reaction. The area should become visibly red, but do not break the skin or induce bleeding.

After the *Gwa Sha*, *Zheng Gu Shui* and *Tieh Ta Yao Gin* have the added benefit of resolving *Blood* stasis that may have been the condition treated in the first place. They can dispel any *Blood* stasis in the form of bruising that may have resulted from the technique. Cupping over the area that was treated with *Gwa Sha* is another common combined Chinese modality.

Never do *Gwa Sha* over an open wound, sore, scar, skin eruptions, ulcerations, or on contagious skin rashes or skin allergies. Do not use on the abdomen of pregnant women. Do not use in case of high fever, bleeding diseases, loose skin, hairy patches, or articulations. Do not use on hypertensive patients, those in a coma. The spoon must be sterilized for each new patient. If other scraping instruments are used, they, too, should be sterilized or, if they are disposable, disposed of properly.

Treating these unique patterns of *Blood* stasis with the techniques described herein is not just a symptomatic treatment of the disorder. Rather, it is a root approach that invigorates stagnant *Qi* and *Blood*, and thus addresses the underlying etiology. The way patients handle their emotions should be pointed out to them so they can recognize how they are expressing their feelings through their bodies. In cases of blood pressure problems, patients should use Western medical techniques in addition to Oriental methods.

Summary

Bloodletting, plum blossom needling, and *Gwa Sha* are powerful therapeutic modalities. Know when and how to use them as well as their contraindications.

Conclusion: Nourishing the Foundation, the Beginning of Health

A benchmark of Oriental medicine has always been its recognition that a person is an individual and a unique pattern of energy that needs to be addressed when they are ill to bring them back to balance and health. This distinct feature is important and yet sometimes it has led to a more symptomatic approach to treatment. The premise of this book has been to achieve a balance between the individuating manifestations of a person's illness with the Chinese recognition that the human body is but *Qi* and *Blood* and essential substances which when ill are for the preponderance of the time deficient and in need of support. The foundational approach to Oriental medical treatment cannot be overlooked and should be part of the practitioner's repertoire of treatment.

At some point, your patients will be released from your care, hopefully physically better as in the case of relief from the common cold or the suffering of the flu. Ideally, they are even emotionally and spiritually better than when they first came to you for treatment since the body and mind are inseparable. For more complex problems, such as chronic back pain or a sequel to stroke, when they leave is something they decide on, or ideally when you can both mutually determine depending on the assessment of their prognosis. They may leave cured, but in a humane system of healthcare ethics, they must leave comforted and healed according to the definition of those terms this book has discussed if one is practicing medicine spiritually, ethically, and "foundationally."

A Tibetan analogy compares the body and the mind (spirit/*Shen*) to a teacup and the tea. The body is like a cup that holds the tea. It is the external form. Like the body, the cup can break and is no longer a cup. The tea, however, like the mind/spirit, remains as tea. Whether the tea is in the cup, spilled on the floor, and absorbed by a rag, it is still tea. It is the essence for which the cup was made. We need to remember that the illness of the body is just a problem with the cup that we do want to care for and cherish like precious china. However, it is just a cup. We need to think beyond the form and savor the essence of the tea/mind/spirit.

This book has been written to prod you as a practitioner into thinking about the broader context of your practice as a healer by treating the foundational energy of the patient. The expectation and clinical results bear out that more long-lasting results can be achieved because that deep foundational energy has been accessed and supplemented.

But additionally, the essential philosophy of this book encourages your presence in the therapeutic encounter. We all have the innate capacity to heal the human spirit. With our hands, our hearts, and minds we can be a presence that listens, supports, comforts, and cures. Medical training is of course an advantage on the physical level, but as we have seen, it is just one dimension of healing. Never underestimate the power that you have as a practitioner to shape the patient's experience of their illness. We need to emulate the fullness of our humanity as a physician, and bring to the healing process not just our knowledge of medicine, herbs, needles, drugs, massage or any other tool, but the richness of our humanity, that includes our spirit, to deal with the pain, suffering, death, illness, healing, and curing of our patient by recognizing their spirit.

It is imperative that if such topics are not presented in school or were not part of your education that you should consider them now. Hopefully through this book and the clinical applications in certain chapters, you will see that your actions have consequence, logic, thought, and purpose.

So be a healing presence for your patients whom you have nourished in their foundational energies. We can all be, genuinely and simply, a human being reaching out to another with great healing effect.

Glossary

Ah Shi   Literally means "Oh, yes." These are points that are tender or sensitive when palpated. They do not have definite locations or names

Bao Gong   The palace or envelope of the child, that is, the uterus

Bao Luo   An internal vessel that connects the Kidney to the uterus

Bao Mai   An internal vessel that connects the Pericardium to the uterus

Baxie   A set of points located on the dorsum of the hands between each finger at the junction of the margins of the webs

Chong Mai   One of the Eight Curious Vessels, the Sea of Blood

Coalescent points   Points of intersection between the twelve regular channels and the Eight Curious Vessels

Confluent points   The Master points that connect the Eight Curious Vessels with the twelve regular meridians and activate the Curious Vessel

Dai Mai   One of the Eight Curious Vessels, the Belt Vessel

Dan Tian   The area in the lower abdomen below the umbilicus that pertains to the Kidney, the root of *Qi*

Da Qi   The sensation of the arrival of *Qi* to the needle

Erjian   The ear apex point

Essential substances   *Qi, Blood, Yin, Yang, Jin-ye, Shen, Marrow*

Foundational energy   *Qi, Blood, Jing, Jin-ye, Shen, Marrow, Yin, Yang,* and *Zang-fu* energies

Gwa Sha   A scraping technique with similar results to bloodletting for the removal of stagnation

Huatojiaji   points A group of points on both sides of the spinal column at the lateral borders of the spinous processes of the first thoracic to the fifth lumbar vertebrae

Jiao   Heater, warmer, burning space

Jing   Rarefied essence, one of the essential substances

Jinjin   One of the veins on the underside of the tongue, located on the frenulum

Jin-ye   The pure fluids retained by the body for its own use

Jueyin   One of the Six Divisions, the lesser *Yin*

Liu Wei Di Huang Wan   Six Flavor Tea, a classical formula for nourishing Kidney and Liver *Yin Hang Wan* deficiency

Luo   Vessel or channel, also a type of point

Mai   Meridian, blood vessel. Sometimes transliterated as *Mo* means channel or vessel

Mu   One of the twelve points on the front of the body that pertain to each of the twelve *Zang-fu* organs

Neijing   The oldest body of Chinese medical literature. Also referred to as *The Yellow Emperor's Classic, The Canon of Acupuncture, The Compendium of Acupuncture and Moxibustion*

Possom On   External Chinese medicated ointment that warms the muscles. Good for aches and pains due to injury, stagnant *Blood* or wind-cold

Qi   Vital energy, the life force

San Jiao   The Triple Warmer, the Triple Heater, the Triple Burner, the Triple Energizer

Shaoyang   The level of the Six Divisions that represents the hinge between the interior and the exterior pertaining to the Gall Bladder and the Triple Burner

Shaoyin   One of the deepest levels of the Six Divisions pertaining to the Heart and Kidney

Shen   Spirit

Shi   Dampness

Shixuan   A group of points on the tips of the ten fingers

Shu   A type of point located on the back medial Bladder line that is associated with the *Qi* of each of the twelve *Zang-fu* organs, as well as other structures

Sifeng   On the palmar surface of the hand at the midpoint of the transverse crease of the interphalangeal joints of the index, middle, ring, and little fingers

Taiyang   The first level of the Six Divisions pertaining to the Bladder and the Small Intestine

Taiyin   The fourth level of the Six Divisions pertaining to Lung and Spleen

Tieh Ta   External Chinese liniment well known for resolving bruises

Wan Hua   External Chinese liniment to move *Blood* stagnation

Wei Qi   Protective, defensive *Qi*

Xi   (cleft)Point of accumulation or blockage

Xie Qi   Pathogenic energy, evil *Qi*

Xin Bao   Pericardium, the envelope that protects the Heart

Xu   Deficiency

Xue   Originally meaning a cave or a hole, which later became a reference for an acupuncture point; or *Blood*

Yangming   One of the Six Division levels, resplendent sunlight

Yangqiao   One of the Eight Curious Vessels, the *Yang* heel vessel

Yangwei   One of the Eight Curious Vessels, the *Yang* connecting vessel

Ying   Nutritive *Qi*

Yinqiao Mai   One of the Eight Curious Vessels, the *Yin* heel vessel

Yinwei   One of the Eight Curious Vessels, the *Yin* linking channel

Yuan Qi   Source *Qi*, reproductive *Qi*, congenital *Qi*, *Qi* of preheaven, original *Qi*, Kidney *Qi*

Yuyue   One of the veins on the underside of the tongue on the frenulum

Zang-fu   The twelve organs in Chinese medicine

Zheng Gu Shui   A powerful external Chinese liniment that penetrates to the bone level and activates *Qi* and *Blood*

References

Beinfield, H. and Korngold, E. (May 1998) 'Eastern medicine for western people.' *Alternative Therapies 4*, 3.

Cohen, J. (October 6, 2010) 'Judaism, health and wholeness.' ABC Religion and Ethics. http://www.abc.net.au/religion/articles/2010/10/06/3030788.htm

County Health Rankings and Roadmaps http://www.countryhealthrankings.org/using-the-rankings-data/broaden-your-view.

Cheng, X. (1999).' Miraculous pivot.' In Cheng X, chief editor. *Chinese Acupuncture and Moxibustion*. Beijing: China Foreign Language Press.

Dale, R.A. (1994) 'Acupuncture needling: a summary of the principal traditional Chinese methods.' *American Journal of Acupuncture*, 22, 2, 167.

Dobb, E. (February 1995) 'Return of the GP.' *Longevity Magazine 74*, 92.

Dossey, L. (2002) 'How healing happens; exploring the nonlocal gap.' *Alternative Therapies 8*, 12.

Flaws, B. (1990) 'The pill and stagnant blood: the side-effects of oral contraceptives according to traditional Chinese medicine.' *Journal of Chinese Medicine 32*, 19–21.

Goleman, D. (1991) Mole quoted in 'Comfort is potent medicine, new research confirms.' *Quintessence* 11–13.

Greenwood, M. (1999) 'Energetics and transformation—insight on the paradoxical opportunity presented by chronic illness and pain—part iiii.' *American Journal of Acupuncture 27*,1/2, 51–56.

Jarrett, L. (1998) *Nourishing Destiny*. Stockbridge, MA: Spirit Path Press.

Kaptchuk, T. (1983) *The Web That Has No Weaver*. New York: Congdon and Weed.

Kelting, T. (1995) 'The nature of nature.' *Parabola XX*, I, 24–30.

Konner, M. (1987) *Becoming a Doctor, A Journey of Initiation in Medical School*. New York: Penguin Press.

Larre, C. and Rochat de la Vallee, E. (Winter 1990–1991) 'The practitioner–patient relationship.' *Journal of Traditional Acupuncture* 14–17 and 48–50.

Larre, C. and Rochat de la Vallee, E. (1995) *Rooted in Spirit.* New York: Station Hill Press.

Maciocia, G. (1989) *The Foundations of Chinese Medicine.* London: Churchill Livingstone.

Matsumoto, K. (1986) *Extraordinary Meridians.* Brookline, MA: Paradigm Publications.

Matsumoto, K. (July 1988) 'Workshop on palpation.' Southwest Acupuncture College, Santa Fe, NM.

Nagai-Jacobson, M. and Burkhardt, M. (2002) 'Story telling: talking to your healthcare practitioner.' *Alternative Therapies 2,* 1, 18–19.

Requena, Y. (1989) *Character and Health: The Relationship of Acupuncture and Psychology.* Brookline, MA: Paradigm Publications.

Rubik, B. (September 1995) 'Can western science provide a foundation for acupuncture?' *Alternative Therapies 1,* 4, 41–47.

Shanghai College of Traditional Chinese Medicine (1981) *Acupuncture: A Comprehensive Text.* Trans. and ed. D. Bensky and J. O'Connor. Chicago: Eastland Press.

Unschuld, P. (1985) *Medicine in China: A History of Ideas.* Berkeley, CA: University of California Press.

Van Nghi, N. (September 1986) 'Luo point use in traditional Chinese medicine.' Lecture. Southwest Acupuncture College, Santa Fe, NM.

Van Nghi, N. (September 1987) 'An exploration of the eight curious vessels.' Lecture. Southwest Acupuncture College, Santa Fe, NM.

Wenbing, Fu and Zhang (2000) 'Contemplation of the treatment of cancerous pain by acupuncture.' *TCM Shanghai Journal of Acupuncture and Moxibustion, English Edition 3,* 57–60.

Wiseman, N., Ellis, A. (trans.) and Zmiewski, P. (ed) (1985) *Fundamentals of Chinese Medicine.* Brookline, MA: Paradigm Press.

World Health Organization (1993) *Standard Acupuncture Nomenclature.* Ed. Regional Office for the Western Pacific. Manila: WHO Regional Office for the Western Pacific.

List of Points

LUNG MERIDIAN

LU 1 Zhongfu

LU 2 Yunmen

LU 3 Tianfu

LU 4 Xiabai

LU 5 Chize

LU 6 Kongzui

LU 7 Lieque

LU 8 Jingqu

LU 9 Taiyuan

LU 10 Yuji

LU 11 Shaoshang

LARGE INTESTINE MERIDIAN

LI 1 Shangyang

LI 2 Erjian

LI 3 Sanjian

LI 4 Hegu

LI 5 Yangxi

LI 6 Pianli

LI 7 Wenliu

LI 8 Xialian

LI 9 Shanglian

LI 10 Shousanli

LI 11 Quchi

LI 12 Zhouliao

LI 13 Shouwuli

LI 14 Binao

LI 15 Jianyu

LI 16 Jugu

LI 17 Tianding

LI 18 Futu

LI 19 Kouheliao

LI 20 Yingxiang

STOMACH MERIDIAN

ST 1 Chengqi

ST 2 Sibai

ST 3 Juliao

ST 4 Dicang

ST 5 Daying

ST 6 Jiache

ST 7 Xiaguan

ST 8 Touwei

ST 9 Renying

ST 10 Shuitu

ST 11 Qishe

ST 12 Quepen

ST 13 Qihu

ST 14 Kufang

ST 15 Wuyi

ST 16 Yingchuang

ST 17 Ruzhong

ST 18 Rugen

ST 19 Burong

ST 20 Chengman

ST 21 Liangmen

ST 22 Guanmen

ST 23 Taiyi

ST 24 Huaroumen

ST 25 Tianshu

ST 26 Wailing

ST 27 Daju

ST 28 Shuidao

ST 29 Guilai

ST 30 Qichong

ST 31 Biguan

ST 32 Futu

ST 33 Yinshi

ST 34 Liangqui

ST 35 Dubi

ST 36 Zusanli

ST 37 Shanjuxu

ST 38 Tiaokou

ST 39 Xiajuxu

ST 40 Fenglong

ST 41 Jiexi

ST 42 Chongyang

ST 43 Xiangu

ST 44 Neiting

ST 45 Lidui

SPLEEN MERIDIAN

SP 1 Yinbai

SP 2 Dadu

SP 3 Taibai

SP 4 Gongsun

SP 5 Shangqiu

SP 6 Sanyinjiao

SP 7 Lougu

SP 8 Diji

SP 9 Yinlingquan

SP 10 Xuehai

SP 11 Jimen

SP 12 Chongmen

SP 13 Fushe

SP 14 Fujie

SP 15 Daheng

SP 16 Fuai

SP 17 Shidou

SP 18 Tianxi

SP 19 Xiongxiang

SP 20 Zhourong

SP 21 Dabao

HEART MERIDIAN

HT 1 Jiquan

HT 2 Qingling

HT 3 Shaohai

HT 4 Lingdao

HT 5 Tongli

HT 6 Yinxi

HT 7 Shenmen

HT 8 Shaofu

HT 9 Shaochong

SMALL INTESTINE MERIDIAN

SI 1 Shaoze

SI 2 Qiangu

SI 3 Houxi

SI 4 Wangu

SI 5 Yanggu

SI 6 Yanglao

SI 7 Zhizheng

SI 8 Xiaohai

SI 9 Jianzhen

SI 10 Noashu

SI 11 Tianzong

SI 12 Bingfeng

SI 13 Quyuan

SI 14 Jianwaishu

SI 15 Jianzhongshu

SI 16 Tianchuang

SI 17 Tianrong

SI 18 Quanliao

SI 19 Tinggong

BLADDER MERIDIAN

BL 1 Jingming

BL 2 Zanzhu

BL 3 Meichong

BL 4 Quchai

BL 5 Wuchu

BL 6 Chengguang

BL 7 Tontian

BL 8 Luoque

BL 9 Yushen

BL 10 Tianzhu

BL 11 Dazhu

BL 12 Fengmen

BL 13 Feishu

BL 14 Jueyinshu

BL 15 Xinshu

BL 16 Dushu

BL 17 Geshu

BL 18 Ganshu

BL 19 Danshu

BL 20 Pishu

BL 21 Weishu

BL 22 Sanjiaoshu

BL 23 Shenshu

BL 24 Qihaishu

BL 25 Dachangshu

BL 26 Guanyuanshu

Bl 27 Xiaochangshu

BL 28 Pangguangshu

BL 29 Zhonglushu

BL 30 Baihuanshu

BL 31 Shangliao

BL 32 Ciliao

BL 33 Zhongliao

BL 34 Xialiao

BL 35 Huiyang

BL 36 Chengfu

BL 37 Yinmen

BL 38 Fuxi

BL 39 Weiyang

BL 40 Weizhong

BL 41 Fufen

BL 42 Pohu

BL 43 Gaohuang

BL 44 Shentang

BL 45 Yixi

BL 46 Geguan

BL 47 Hunmen

BL 48 Yanggang

BL 49 Yishe

BL 50 Weicang

BL 51 Huangmen

BL 52 Zhishi

BL 53 Baohuang

BL 54 Zhibian

BL 55 Heyang

BL 56 Chengjin

BL 57 Chengshan

BL 58 Feiyang

BL 59 Fuyang

BL 60 Kunlun

BL 61 Pucan

BL 62 Shenmai

BL 63 Jinmen

BL 64 Jinggu

BL 65 Shugu

BL 66 Zutonggu

BL 67 Zhiyin

KIDNEY MERIDIAN

KI 1 Yongquan

KI 2 Rangu

KI 3 Taixi

KI 4 Dazhong

KI 5 Shuiquan

KI 6 Zhaohai

KI 7 Fuliu

KI 8 Jiaoxin

KI 9 Zhubin

KI 10 Yingu

KI 11 Henggu

KI 12 Dahe

KI 13 Qixue

KI 14 Siman

KI 15 Zhongzhu

KI 16 Huangshu

KI 17 Shangqu

KI 18 Shiguan

KI 19 Yindu

KI 20 Futonggu

KI 21 Youmen

KI 22 Bulang

KI 23 Shenfeng

KI 24 Lingxu

KI 25 Shencang

KI 26 Yuzhong

KI 27 Shufu

PERICARDIUM MERIDIAN

PC 1 Tianchi

PC 2 Tianquan

PC 3 Quze

PC 4 Ximen

PC 5 Jianshi

PC 6 Neiguan

PC 7 Daling

PC 8 Laogong

PC 9 Zhongchong

SANJIAO (TRIPLE BURNER) MERIDIAN

TB 1 Guanchong

TB 2 Yemen

TB 3 Zhongdu

TB 4 Yangchi

TB 5 Waiguan

TB 6 Zhigou

TB 7 Huizong

TB 8 Sanyangluo

TB 9 Sidu

TB 10 Tianjing

TB 11 Qinglenzuan

TB 12 Xiaoluo

TB 13 Naohui

TB 14 Jianliao

TB 15 Tianliao

TB 16 Tianyou

TB 17 Yifeng

TB 18 Qimai

TB 19 Luxi

TB 20 Jiaosun

TB 21 Ermen

TB 22 Erheliao

TB 23 Sizhukong

GALL BLADDER MERIDIAN

GB 1 Tongziliao

GB 2 Tinghui

GB 3 Shangguan

GB 4 Hanyan

GB 5 Xuanlu

GB 6 Xuanli

GB 7 Qubin

GB 8 Shuaigu

GB 9 Tianchong

GB 10 Fubai

GB 11 Touqiaoyin

GB 12 Wangu

GB 13 Benshen

GB 14 Yangbai

GB 15 Toulinqi

GB 16 Muchuang

GB 17 Zhengying

GB 18 Chengling

GB 19 Naokong

GB 20 Fengchi

GB 21 Jianjing

GB 22 Yuanye

GB 23 Zhejin

GB 24 Riyue

GB 25 Jingmen

GB 26 Daimai

GB 27 Wushu

GB 28 Weidao

GB 29 Juliao

GB 30 Huantiao

GB 31 Fengshi

GB 32 Zhongdu

GB 33 Xiyangguan

GB 34 Yanglingquan

GB 35 Yangjiao

GB 36 Wauqui

GB 37 Guangming

GB 38 Yangfu

GB 39 Xuanzhong

GB 40 Quixu

GB 41 Zulinqi

GB 42 Diwuhui

GB 43 Xiaxi

GB 44 Zuqiaoyin

LIVER MERIDIAN

LR 1 Dadun

LR 2 Xingjian

LR 3 Taichong

LR 4 Zhongfeng

LR 5 Ligou

LR 6 Zhongdu

LR 7 Xiguan .

LR 8 Ququan

LR 9 Yinbao

LR 10 Zuwuli

LR 11 Yinlian

LR 12 Jimai

LR 13 Zhangmen

LR 14 Qimen

GOVERNING VESSEL

GV 1 Changqiang

GV 2 Yaoshu

GV 3 Yaoyangguan

GV 4 Mingmen

GV 5 Xuanshu

GV 6 Jizhong

GV 7 Zhongshu

GV 8 Jinsuo

GV 9 Zhiyang

GV 10 Lingtai

GV 11 Shendao

GV 12 Shenzhu

GV 13 Taodao

GV 14 Dazhui

GV 15 Yamen

GV 16 Fengfu

GV 17 Noahu

GV 18 Qiangjian

GV 19 Houding

GV 20 Baihui

GV 21 Qianding

GV 22 Xinhui

GV 23 Shangxin

GV 24 Shenting

GV 25 Suliao

GV 26 Shuigou

GV 27 Duiduan

GV 28 Yinjiao

CONCEPTION VESSEL

CV 1 Huiyin

CV 2 Qugu

CV 3 Zhongji

CV 4 Guanyuan

CV 5 Shimen

CV 6 Qihai

CV 7 Yinjiao

CV 8 Shenque

CV 9 Shuifen

CV 10 Xiawan

CV 11 Jianli

CV 12 Zhongwan

CV 13 Shangwan

CV 14 Juque

CV 15 Jiuwei

CV 16 Zhongting

CV 17 Tanzhong

CV 18 Yutang

CV 19 Zigong

CV 20 Huagai

CV 21 Xuanji

CV 22 Tiantu

CV 23 Lianquan

CV 24 Chengjiang

Index

About the Author

Skya Abbate, DOM (Doctor of Oriental Medicine), Dipl Ac, Dipl CH, MA Sociology, MPS Pastoral Studies and MA Bioethics and Health Policy

Skya began her career as a medical sociologist serving as a Peace Corps volunteer in Brazil and then later taught in the Sociology Department of the University of Rhode Island from 1978-1981. She holds a B.A. in Sociology from Salve Regina College Newport, RI (1973), where she graduated *summa cum laude* and class valedictorian, and an M. A. in Sociology from the University of Rhode Island conferred in 1978.

Following pre-med studies at the University of Rhode Island (1983), Skya graduated from the acupuncture program of the Institute of Traditional Medicine in Santa Fe, NM. She then undertook two advanced clinical training programs with the Academy of Traditional Chinese Medicine in Beijing, China in 1988 and 1989. She also holds a Masters degree in Pastoral Studies (Loyola University New Orleans, 2012) and a Masters degree in Bioethics and Health Policy (Loyola University Chicago, 2016). Currently she is enrolled in the doctoral program in Public Health and Catholic Bioethics with Loyola University, Chicago.

Skya is a licensed Doctor of Oriental Medicine in the state of New Mexico, Executive Director of Southwest Acupuncture College with campuses in Santa Fe, NM and Boulder, CO. She was former President of the New Mexico Association of Acupuncture and Oriental Medicine and has served for over six years as an educational expert and Commissioner for the Accreditation Commission for Schools and Colleges of Acupuncture and Oriental Medicine (ACAOM), the national organization that accredits professional degree programs in Oriental medicine.

Skya is the author of seventeen books in numerous genres from medicine to liturgy, poetry, and history, illustrated children's stories, and close to forty published articles in acupuncture journals and one in bioethics published in such prestigious journals as the *American Journal of Acupuncture*, the *Journal of Chinese Medicine*, the *New England Journal of Traditional Chinese Medicine*, and *Acupuncture Today* where she served for six years as the needle technique columnist.

With over thirty years of private practice, teaching, and writing in Oriental medicine, she is one of the most respected and prolific women writers in Oriental medicine in the Western world. Skya teaches needle technique, diagnosis, and Japanese acupuncture systems at Southwest Acupuncture College. She lives in Santa Fe, New Mexico with her husband of over thirty years. She raises exotic goldfish and study birds daily and loves everything about fish and birds!

CPI Antony Rowe
Eastbourne, UK
February 16, 2022